Table of Contents

Foreword

Welcome to "Balanced Brain, Balanced Body: Nutrition and Supplements for Mental Health." This book is your gateway to understanding the profound connection between what you eat and how you feel. In today's fast-paced world, where stress and anxiety often feel like constant companions, it's essential to recognize the power of nutrition in transforming our mental well-being.

Imagine a life where your mind feels as nourished and balanced as your body. A diet rich in essential nutrients like vitamins, minerals, and omega-3 fatty acids can be a game-changer, significantly impacting your mental health. Scientific research has repeatedly shown that the right nutrients and supplements can play a pivotal role in managing stress, anxiety, and depression, as well as enhancing cognitive function.

Dive into the fascinating world of nutritional supplements and discover how they can help reduce stress and anxiety. Minerals such as magnesium, essential B vitamins, and zinc have been proven to alleviate these symptoms, promoting a calmer state of mind. Herbal supplements like ashwagandha and rhodiola offer additional natural support, helping to soothe and balance both body and mind. Incorporating these powerful supplements into your daily routine can dramatically enhance your mental well-being.

Whether your goal is to manage stress, sharpen your cognitive abilities, or lift the weight of depression, the right combination of nutrients and supplements can make a world of difference. This book will guide you through the essentials of prioritizing your nutritional intake, offering practical advice and insights to help you maintain a healthy mind and body for years to come.

Prepare to embark on a journey towards mental clarity and emotional balance. "Balanced Brain, Balanced Body" is more than just a guide; it's your companion in achieving optimal mental health through the power of nutrition. Let's unlock the secrets to a vibrant, healthier you.

How Nutritional Deficiencies Can Impact Mental Health

Nutritional deficiencies can profoundly impact your mental health, often silently disrupting your well-being. When your body lacks essential nutrients, imbalances in neurotransmitters, hormones, and other chemicals that regulate mood, stress, and cognitive function can occur. These imbalances may lead to anxiety, depression, fatigue, and poor concentration, which you might mistakenly attribute solely to external factors like stress or lifestyle choices.

In our modern society, where processed foods are abundant and nutrient-dense foods are often overlooked, it's crucial to pay attention to your nutritional intake. The convenience of fast food and pre-packaged meals often comes at the expense of essential vitamins and minerals, leaving your brain and body starved of what they need to function optimally. Understanding which nutrients are vital and how their deficiencies can impact mental health is the first step towards reclaiming your well-being.

For instance, a lack of B vitamins can lead to mood swings and cognitive decline, while insufficient magnesium levels are linked to increased stress and anxiety. Iron deficiency can cause fatigue and impair cognitive function, and a shortage of omega-3 fatty acids can exacerbate depression and mood disorders. By recognizing these deficiencies and incorporating the right foods and supplements into your diet, you can restore balance and support your mental health.

Importance of Balancing Nutrient Levels for Mental Health

Before exploring the benefits of herbs and nootropics, it's crucial to understand that the most important step in addressing mental health issues is to ensure that your body has the essential nutrients it needs. Nutrient imbalances can significantly disrupt both physical and mental health, leading to a wide range of issues that herbs and nootropics alone cannot address.

Physical Health: When the body lacks essential nutrients, it can lead to various health problems. Nutrient imbalances can weaken the immune system, making you more susceptible to infections and diseases. It can also affect your energy levels, leading to chronic fatigue and a decreased ability to perform daily tasks. Other physical symptoms can include muscle weakness, bone pain, and cardiovascular issues, all of which stem from the body's inability to function optimally without the necessary nutrients.

Mental Health: The brain is particularly sensitive to nutrient imbalances. Essential nutrients play a crucial role in neurotransmitter function, the chemical messengers that regulate mood, cognition, and overall mental well-being. A deficiency in these nutrients can lead to mood swings, anxiety, depression, and cognitive impairments such as poor memory and concentration. The brain's inability to produce and regulate neurotransmitters effectively can exacerbate mental health issues, creating a vicious cycle of deteriorating mental health.

Restoring Balance: To restore balance and support both mental and physical health, it's imperative to identify and correct any nutrient deficiencies. This often involves a comprehensive approach that includes blood tests to determine specific deficiencies, followed by dietary adjustments and supplementation under the guidance of a healthcare professional. Ensuring that your body receives the right balance of vitamins, minerals, and other essential nutrients lays the foundation for overall health and well-being.

In This chapter will explore the most prevalent nutritional deficiencies, their impacts on both mental and overall health, and offer practical dietary solutions. From leafy greens and fatty fish to nuts and seeds, you'll discover how to nourish your body and mind effectively. Join us on this journey to uncover the powerful connection between nutrition and mental well-being, and learn how to create a balanced, nutrient-rich diet that supports a healthy, happy mind.

Vitamin D Deficiency

Vitamin D is a crucial nutrient that plays a fundamental role in both mental and physical health. Understanding the effects of vitamin D deficiency and ensuring adequate intake through diet, sunlight exposure, and supplements is essential for maintaining overall well-being.

Effect on Mental Health

Vitamin D deficiency can significantly impact mental health by affecting neurotransmitter function and mood regulation.

- *Depression and Anxiety:* Low levels of vitamin D have been associated with increased symptoms of depression and anxiety. Vitamin D receptors are present in areas of the brain involved in mood regulation, and deficiency may disrupt neurotransmitter pathways.

- *Seasonal Affective Disorder (SAD):* Vitamin D deficiency is linked to seasonal affective disorder, a type of depression that occurs during specific seasons, often in the winter months when sunlight exposure is limited. Sunlight triggers the production of vitamin D in the skin, and decreased sunlight can lead to lower vitamin D levels and worsening symptoms of depression.

Effect on Overall Health

Vitamin D is essential for various bodily functions beyond mental health, including bone health, immune function, and cardiovascular health.

- *Bone Health:* Vitamin D plays a critical role in calcium absorption and bone mineralization. Deficiency can lead to weakened bones, increasing the risk of fractures and osteoporosis.

- *Immune Function:* Adequate vitamin D levels are necessary for a healthy immune system. Vitamin D helps regulate immune cell activity and promotes the production of antimicrobial peptides that defend against infections.

- *Cardiovascular Health:* Vitamin D deficiency is associated with an increased risk of cardiovascular diseases, including hypertension, heart attack, and stroke. Vitamin D helps regulate blood pressure and reduce inflammation in the cardiovascular system.

Supplements

Ensuring adequate vitamin D intake through supplements can be beneficial, especially for individuals who have limited sunlight exposure or are at risk of deficiency.

- *Vitamin D Supplements:* These are available in various forms, including vitamin D3 (cholecalciferol) and vitamin D2 (ergocalciferol). The recommended daily intake of vitamin D varies by age, sex, and health status but generally ranges from 600 to 800 IU (International Units) per day for adults.

- *Supplement Forms:* Vitamin D supplements come in pills, capsules, drops, and even chewable forms. It's essential to choose a form that is well-absorbed by the body, such as vitamin D3.

- *Dosage and Absorption:* The dosage of vitamin D supplements may need to be adjusted based on individual factors such as age, ethnicity, and geographic location. It's also important to take vitamin D supplements with food containing fat to enhance absorption.

Nutrition and Vegetables and Fruit Which Contains the Vitamin or Other Biological Element

While vitamin D is primarily synthesized in the skin through sunlight exposure, some foods contain small amounts of vitamin D.

- *Fatty Fish:* Salmon, mackerel, tuna, and sardines are excellent sources of vitamin D. A serving of fatty fish can provide a significant portion of your daily vitamin D needs.

- *Fortified Foods:* Many foods are fortified with vitamin D, including milk, orange juice, cereal, and yogurt. These fortified foods can help contribute to your overall vitamin D intake, especially for individuals who have limited sunlight exposure.

- *Egg Yolks:* Egg yolks contain small amounts of vitamin D. Including eggs in your diet can provide additional vitamin D, along with other essential nutrients.

- *Mushrooms:* Some varieties of mushrooms, such as shiitake and portobello mushrooms, contain vitamin D when exposed to sunlight during growth. Including mushrooms in your diet can offer a plant-based source of vitamin D.

But the best remedy against lack of vitamin D is ... Sunshine!

The Importance of Sunlight for Vitamin D Production

One of the most effective remedies against vitamin D deficiency is ensuring adequate exposure to natural sunlight. Our bodies have an incredible ability to produce vitamin D when our skin is exposed to ultraviolet B (UVB) rays from the sun. Just a small amount of sun exposure can trigger this process, making sunlight a powerful, natural source of this essential nutrient.

How Much Sunlight Do You Need?

The amount of sunlight needed to produce sufficient vitamin D can vary based on several factors, including geographic location, skin type, age, and the time of year. For most people, exposing the face, arms, or legs to sunlight for about 10 to 30 minutes several times a week is typically sufficient. Those with darker skin may require slightly longer exposure due to higher melanin levels, which can reduce the skin's ability to produce vitamin D. Conversely, individuals with lighter skin may need less time in the sun.

Seasonal Considerations

In regions with distinct seasons, sunlight exposure can vary significantly. During winter months, especially in higher latitudes, the sun's angle may not provide enough UVB rays for vitamin D production. During these times, it's essential to seek alternative sources of vitamin D, such as supplements and vitamin D-rich foods, to maintain adequate levels.

Incorporating Sunlight into Your Routine

Finding time for regular sunlight exposure can be simple and enjoyable. Here are some ideas to incorporate sunlight into your daily routine:

- *Morning Walks:* Start your day with a short walk outside to enjoy the morning sun.
- *Outdoor Activities:* Engage in outdoor activities like gardening, cycling, or playing sports to increase your sun exposure.
- *Lunch Breaks:* Spend your lunch break outside when possible, even if it's just for a few minutes.
- *Sunlit Spaces:* Create sunlit spaces in your home or workplace where you can sit and soak up the rays during the day.

Balancing Sunlight with Other Sources of Vitamin D

While sunlight is a powerful source of vitamin D, it's crucial to complement it with dietary sources and supplements, especially during periods of limited sun exposure. This balanced approach ensures you maintain optimal vitamin D levels year-round, supporting not only your bone health but also your emotional well-being. However, be cautious—vitamin D overdose is harmful, so it's essential to stick to the prescribed dosage.

As we move forward, we'll explore another critical nutrient that could be silently impacting your mental and physical health. Just as vitamin D plays a pivotal role in your body, so too do other essential vitamins and minerals. Stay tuned as we delve into the next vital nutrient and uncover simple, actionable steps to enhance your health and vitality!

Omega-3 Fatty Acids Imbalance

Omega-3 fatty acids are essential fats that play a critical role in maintaining both mental and physical health. An imbalance or deficiency in omega-3s can have profound effects, making it crucial to understand their importance and how to incorporate them into your diet effectively.

Effect on Mental Health

Omega-3 fatty acids, particularly eicosapentaenoic acid (EPA) and docosahexaenoic acid (DHA), are vital for brain health. These essential fats are integral components of cell membranes in the brain and influence cell signaling pathways.

- *Depression and Anxiety:* Low levels of omega-3s have been associated with increased symptoms of depression and anxiety. Studies have shown that individuals who consume higher amounts of omega-3s tend to have lower rates of these mental health conditions.

- *Cognitive Function:* Omega-3s are crucial for cognitive development and function. Deficiencies can lead to difficulties with memory, focus, and overall cognitive performance. In children, adequate omega-3 intake is linked to better learning and behavior outcomes.

Effect on Overall Health

Beyond mental health, omega-3 fatty acids contribute to various aspects of overall health.

- *Cardiovascular Health:* Omega-3s are known to reduce inflammation, lower blood pressure, and decrease the risk of heart disease. They help maintain a healthy heart rhythm and reduce the likelihood of heart attacks and strokes.

- *Inflammatory Diseases:* These fatty acids have anti-inflammatory properties that can help manage conditions like arthritis and inflammatory bowel disease (IBD). Regular intake can reduce the severity and frequency of flare-ups.

Supplements

To ensure adequate intake of omega-3s, supplements can be a practical option, especially for those who do not consume enough through their diet.

- *Fish Oil Supplements:* These are one of the most common sources of omega-3s, providing a substantial amount of EPA and DHA. It is generally recommended to take 1,000 to 2,000 mg per day, depending on individual health needs and dietary intake.

- *Algal Oil Supplements:* For vegetarians and vegans, algal oil is an excellent alternative to fish oil, offering a plant-based source of DHA.

- *Daily Intake Recommendations:* The American Heart Association suggests eating at least two servings of fatty fish per week, which equates to about 500 mg of EPA and DHA per day for general health. For specific health concerns, higher doses may be recommended under medical supervision.

Nutrient-Rich Foods

While omega-3 fatty acids are predominantly found in animal sources, certain plant-based foods also contain them, particularly alpha-linolenic acid (ALA), which the body can partially convert to EPA and DHA.

- *Fatty Fish:* Salmon, mackerel, sardines, and trout are excellent sources of EPA and DHA. Including these in your diet twice a week can help maintain healthy omega-3 levels.

- *Plant-Based Sources:* Flaxseeds, chia seeds, and walnuts are rich in ALA. Including these in your diet can provide a good source of omega-3s, especially for those following a plant-based diet.

- *Vegetables:* While vegetables are not primary sources of omega-3s, some, like Brussels sprouts and spinach, contain small amounts of ALA and contribute to overall nutrient intake.

- *Fortified Foods:* Certain foods, such as eggs, milk, and yogurt, are fortified with omega-3s and can help boost intake, especially for those who may not consume enough fish or plant-based sources.

B Vitamins Deficiency

B vitamins are a group of water-soluble vitamins that play vital roles in maintaining optimal brain function and overall health. Deficiencies in B vitamins can have severe consequences, making it crucial to understand their importance and ensure adequate intake through diet and supplements.

Effect on Mental Health

B vitamins, including B1 (thiamine), B2 (riboflavin), B3 (niacin), B6 (pyridoxine), B9 (folate), and B12 (cobalamin), are essential for mental health. They help in the synthesis of neurotransmitters, which are critical for mood regulation and cognitive function.

- *Depression:* Low levels of B12 and folate are linked to increased risk of depression. These vitamins are involved in the production of serotonin and dopamine, neurotransmitters that regulate mood.

- *Cognitive Decline:* Deficiencies in B6, B12, and folate can lead to cognitive impairments, including memory loss and decreased concentration. B12 deficiency, in particular, is associated with an increased risk of dementia and Alzheimer's disease.

- *Anxiety and Irritability:* Inadequate levels of B1 and B6 can contribute to anxiety and irritability. These vitamins play a role in the nervous system function and stress response.

Effect on Overall Health

B vitamins are not only crucial for mental health but also for various bodily functions and overall health.

- *Energy Production:* B vitamins, especially B1, B2, B3, and B6, are essential for converting food into energy. Deficiencies can lead to fatigue and weakness.

- *Red Blood Cell Formation:* Vitamins B6, B9, and B12 are vital for the production and maintenance of red blood cells. A deficiency can cause anemia, leading to symptoms like fatigue, shortness of breath, and dizziness.

- *Metabolic Function:* B vitamins support metabolism by helping the body break down carbohydrates, fats, and proteins. A deficiency can disrupt metabolic processes and lead to weight gain or loss and other metabolic disorders.

Supplements

To prevent deficiencies, taking B vitamin supplements can be beneficial, especially for individuals with dietary restrictions or certain health conditions.

- *B Complex Supplements:* These supplements contain all eight B vitamins and are a convenient way to ensure adequate intake. The recommended daily intake varies, but a typical B complex supplement provides about 100% of the daily value for each B vitamin.

- *Individual B Vitamins:* Depending on specific needs, individual B vitamin supplements, such as B12 or folate, can be taken. For example, the recommended daily intake for B12 is about 2.4 micrograms, and for folate, it is about 400 micrograms.

- *Monthly B12 Injections:* For individuals with severe B12 deficiency, monthly injections may be necessary to maintain adequate levels.

Nutrient-Rich Foods

B vitamins are found in a variety of foods, making it possible to meet daily requirements through a balanced diet.

- *Animal Products:* Meat, poultry, fish, eggs, and dairy are rich sources of B12, B6, and niacin. For example, a serving of salmon provides a substantial amount of B12, while chicken and beef are good sources of B6 and niacin.

- *Leafy Greens and Vegetables:* Spinach, kale, broccoli, and Brussels sprouts are excellent sources of folate and riboflavin. Including these vegetables in your diet can help maintain adequate levels of these B vitamins.

- *Legumes and Seeds:* Lentils, chickpeas, and sunflower seeds are rich in B1, B6, and folate. These plant-based foods are especially important for vegetarians and vegans.

- *Fortified Foods:* Many cereals, bread, and plant-based milk are fortified with B vitamins, including B12 and folate, making it easier to meet daily requirements through a varied diet.

Iron Deficiency

Iron deficiency is a common nutritional issue that can have significant impacts on both mental and physical health. Understanding the importance of iron, recognizing its effects, and ensuring adequate intake through diet and supplements is crucial for maintaining overall well-being.

Effect on Mental Health

Iron is essential for proper brain function and mental health. It plays a critical role in the production of neurotransmitters, which are chemicals that transmit signals in the brain.

- *Cognitive Impairment:* Iron deficiency can lead to cognitive issues such as poor concentration, memory problems, and decreased attention span. This is particularly evident in children, where iron deficiency can impair learning and academic performance.

- *Mood Disorders:* Low iron levels are linked to mood disorders, including depression and anxiety. Iron is necessary for the synthesis of dopamine and serotonin, neurotransmitters that regulate mood and emotional well-being.

- *Fatigue and Lethargy:* A lack of iron can cause persistent fatigue and a feeling of lethargy, which can impact daily functioning and overall quality of life.

Effect on Overall Health

Iron is vital for various bodily functions, particularly for the formation of hemoglobin, a protein in red blood cells that carries oxygen throughout the body.

- *Anemia:* Iron deficiency is the most common cause of anemia, characterized by a lack of healthy red blood cells. Symptoms of anemia include fatigue, weakness, pale skin, and shortness of breath.

- *Immune Function:* Adequate iron levels are essential for a healthy immune system. Iron deficiency can impair immune response, making the body more susceptible to infections.

- *Physical Performance:* Iron is crucial for muscle function and endurance. Athletes and individuals engaging in regular physical activity may experience decreased performance and increased fatigue if iron levels are low.

Supplements

Iron supplements can be an effective way to address deficiency, especially for individuals who struggle to get enough iron from their diet alone.

- *Iron Supplements:* These are available in various forms, including ferrous sulfate, ferrous gluconate, and ferrous fumarate. The recommended daily intake of iron varies by age, sex, and health status but generally ranges from 8 to 18 mg per day for adults.

- *Supplement Forms:* Iron supplements can come in pills, capsules, liquid, or even intravenous forms for those with severe deficiencies. It's important to take them as directed, as excessive iron can cause toxicity.

- *Timing and Absorption:* To enhance absorption, iron supplements should be taken on an empty stomach or with vitamin C-rich foods. However, they can cause gastrointestinal discomfort, so some may need to take them with food.

Nutrient-Rich Foods

Iron is present in both animal and plant-based foods, but the type of iron and its absorption rate differ.

- *Animal Sources:* Red meat, poultry, and fish are excellent sources of heme iron, which is more easily absorbed by the body. For instance, beef, liver, and turkey are particularly rich in iron.

- *Plant-Based Sources:* Although non-heme iron from plant sources is less efficiently absorbed, it can still significantly contribute to iron intake. Examples include lentils, chickpeas, tofu, spinach, and fortified cereals.

- *Enhancing Absorption:* Consuming vitamin C-rich foods like oranges, strawberries, bell peppers, and tomatoes alongside iron-rich foods can enhance the absorption of non-heme iron.

- *Foods to Limit:* Certain foods and beverages, such as coffee, tea, dairy products, and foods high in calcium, can inhibit iron absorption and should be consumed at different times from iron-rich meals.

Magnesium Deficiency

Magnesium is an essential mineral that plays a vital role in numerous physiological processes, including those that support mental and physical health. Understanding the effects of magnesium deficiency and ensuring adequate intake through diet and supplements is critical for maintaining overall well-being.

Effect on Mental Health

Magnesium is crucial for brain function and mental health, influencing neurotransmitter activity and brain plasticity.

- *Anxiety and Depression:* Low levels of magnesium are linked to increased symptoms of anxiety and depression. Magnesium helps regulate neurotransmitters like serotonin, which is important for mood stabilization.

- *Stress Response:* Magnesium deficiency can exacerbate the body's response to stress, leading to increased cortisol levels and prolonged periods of anxiety. Adequate magnesium helps modulate the stress response, promoting relaxation and calmness.

- *Cognitive Function:* Magnesium plays a role in cognitive functions such as memory and learning. Deficiency can impair these processes, leading to issues with concentration and mental clarity.

Effect on Overall Health

Magnesium supports numerous bodily functions that are essential for maintaining overall health.

- *Muscle and Nerve Function:* Magnesium is involved in muscle contraction and nerve function. Deficiency can lead to muscle cramps, spasms, and general muscle weakness.

- *Cardiovascular Health:* Adequate magnesium levels are important for maintaining a healthy heart rhythm and preventing cardiovascular diseases. Magnesium deficiency is associated with increased risk of hypertension and heart arrhythmias.

- *Bone Health:* Magnesium is critical for bone health as it helps in the absorption and metabolism of calcium. Deficiency can contribute to osteoporosis and increased fracture risk.

Supplements

Magnesium supplements can be an effective way to address deficiency, especially for individuals who may not get enough from their diet.

- *Magnesium Supplements:* These are available in various forms, including magnesium oxide, magnesium citrate, and magnesium glycinate. The recommended daily intake of magnesium varies by age and sex but generally ranges from 310 to 420 mg per day for adults.

- *Supplement Forms:* Magnesium supplements come in pills, capsules, powders, and even topical forms like oils and lotions. Each form has different absorption rates and benefits.

- *Dosage and Absorption:* It's important to choose a form of magnesium that is well-absorbed by the body. Magnesium citrate and magnesium glycinate are often recommended for their higher bioavailability.

Nutrient-Rich Foods

Magnesium is found in a variety of foods, making it possible to meet daily requirements through a balanced diet.

- *Leafy Greens:* Spinach, kale, and Swiss chard are rich sources of magnesium. Including these greens in your diet can help boost your magnesium intake.

- *Nuts and Seeds:* Almonds, cashews, pumpkin seeds, and sunflower seeds are excellent sources of magnesium. They make for convenient snacks and can be added to salads, yogurts, or smoothies.

- *Whole Grains:* Brown rice, quinoa, and whole wheat bread are good sources of magnesium. Incorporating these grains into meals can contribute to your daily magnesium needs.

- *Legumes:* Black beans, chickpeas, and lentils provide a substantial amount of magnesium. These can be included in soups, stews, and salads.

- *Fruits:* While fruits are not the highest sources of magnesium, some, like bananas, avocados, and figs, can help contribute to your overall intake.

Zinc Deficiency

Zinc is an essential mineral that plays a crucial role in various bodily functions, including immune function, wound healing, and DNA synthesis. Understanding the effects of zinc deficiency and ensuring adequate intake through diet and supplements is essential for maintaining overall well-being.

Effect on Mental Health

Zinc deficiency can impact mental health by affecting neurotransmitter function and brain development.

- *Depression and Anxiety:* Low levels of zinc have been associated with increased symptoms of depression and anxiety. Zinc plays a role in the regulation of neurotransmitters like serotonin and dopamine, which are involved in mood regulation.

- *Cognitive Function:* Zinc is necessary for proper brain development and cognitive function. Deficiency can lead to impaired memory, attention, and learning abilities.

- *Sleep Disturbances:* Zinc deficiency may contribute to sleep disturbances, including insomnia and disrupted sleep patterns. Adequate zinc levels are essential for the production of melatonin, a hormone that regulates sleep.

Effect on Overall Health

Zinc is involved in numerous bodily processes that are crucial for maintaining overall health and well-being.

- *Immune Function:* Zinc is essential for a healthy immune system. It helps support the function of white blood cells and promotes the production of antibodies, which are necessary for fighting infections.

- *Wound Healing:* Zinc plays a critical role in wound healing and tissue repair. It helps in the synthesis of collagen, a protein that is essential for skin health and wound closure.

- *Reproductive Health:* Zinc is important for reproductive health in both men and women. It is involved in the production of sex hormones and sperm production in men.

Supplements

Zinc supplements can be an effective way to address deficiency, especially for individuals who may not get enough from their diet alone.

- *Zinc Supplements:* These are available in various forms, including zinc gluconate, zinc sulfate, and zinc citrate. The recommended daily intake of zinc varies by age and sex but generally ranges from 8 to 11 mg per day for adults.

- *Supplement Forms:* Zinc supplements come in pills, capsules, and lozenges. Some supplements also contain other nutrients like vitamin C, which can enhance zinc absorption.

- *Dosage and Absorption:* It's important to take zinc supplements as directed and to avoid excessive intake, as high doses can interfere with the absorption of other minerals like copper.

Nutrient-Rich Foods

Zinc is found in a variety of foods, making it possible to meet daily requirements through a balanced diet.

- *Animal Sources:* Red meat, poultry, and seafood are rich sources of zinc. For example, a serving of beef provides a significant amount of zinc, while oysters are one of the highest food sources of zinc.

- *Nuts and Seeds:* Pumpkin seeds, hemp seeds, and cashews are good plant-based sources of zinc. These can be enjoyed as snacks or added to salads and stir-fries.

- *Legumes:* Beans, lentils, and chickpeas are also good sources of zinc. Including these legumes in meals can help boost your zinc intake, especially for vegetarians and vegans.

- *Dairy Products:* Dairy foods like milk, cheese, and yogurt contain zinc. These can be incorporated into your diet as part of balanced meals or snacks.

- *Whole Grains:* Whole grains like wheat, oats, and quinoa contain small amounts of zinc. Consuming a variety of whole grains can contribute to your overall zinc intake.

Herbal Supplements

Herbal supplements have been cherished for centuries, playing a pivotal role in traditional medicine to support mental and overall health. These natural remedies, rich in bioactive compounds, can profoundly influence neurotransmitter activity, alleviate stress, and enhance cognitive function. As modern science begins to unravel the mechanisms behind these age-old practices, the potential benefits of herbal supplements for your mental wellbeing are becoming increasingly evident.

In this chapter, we will explore the fascinating world of herbal supplements, exploring 20 of the most effective herbs for treating mental disorders. You'll discover how these herbs work, their historical significance, recommended daily intake, and potential side effects. From the calming effects of ashwagandha to the cognitive-boosting properties of ginkgo biloba, each supplement offers unique benefits that can contribute to a balanced mind and body.

Join us on this journey through nature's pharmacy, where ancient wisdom meets modern research. By understanding the power of these herbal allies, you can make informed choices to support your mental well-being and overall health. Let's explore how these remarkable plants can become a part of your daily routine, providing natural solutions for a healthier, happier life.

Ashwagandha

Ashwagandha, also known as *Withania somnifera*, is a powerful adaptogenic herb originating from India, where it has been used for over 3,000 years in Ayurvedic medicine. Its name translates to "smell of the horse," which reflects its traditional belief to impart the strength and vitality of a stallion. Historically, Indian tribes and Ayurvedic practitioners used ashwagandha to enhance stamina, reduce stress, and promote longevity. It was especially valued for its ability to balance the body's systems and enhance overall well-being.

In modern times, ashwagandha has gained widespread popularity as a natural remedy for stress and anxiety. Numerous studies have supported its efficacy in reducing cortisol levels, the body's primary stress hormone, and improving symptoms of anxiety and depression. Current research also indicates that ashwagandha can enhance cognitive function, boost memory, and support neuroplasticity, making it a valuable ally for mental health. Its adaptogenic properties help the body to adapt to stress and restore balance, which is particularly beneficial in today's fast-paced world.

Today, ashwagandha is widely available in various forms, including capsules, powders, and teas, and is often used as a natural supplement to support mental well-being, improve energy levels, and promote overall health. As science continues to explore its potential, ashwagandha remains a testament to the enduring power of traditional herbal medicine.

Intake:

— 300-500 mg of standardized extract, taken once or twice daily.

Potential Side Effects:

— Stomach upset, drowsiness, and allergic reactions in some individuals.

St. John's Wort

St. John's Wort, scientifically known as *Hypericum perforatum*, is a flowering plant native to Europe, where it has been used medicinally for centuries. Its use dates back to ancient Greece, with notable figures like Hippocrates and Pliny the Elder documenting its healing properties. During the Middle Ages, it was used by various European tribes and cultures to ward off evil spirits and treat wounds, burns, and a variety of ailments. The name "St. John's Wort" comes from its tradition of blooming around St. John's Day, celebrated on June 24th.

In contemporary times, St. John's Wort is primarily recognized for its antidepressant properties. Numerous studies have shown that it can be effective in treating mild to moderate depression, often compared favorably to conventional antidepressants with fewer side effects. The herb contains active compounds such as hypericin and hyperforin, which are believed to enhance neurotransmitter activity, particularly serotonin, dopamine, and norepinephrine, thereby improving mood and emotional balance.

Today, St. John's Wort is widely available as a supplement in the form of capsules, tablets, teas, and tinctures. Its natural antidepressant and anti-inflammatory properties make it a popular choice for those seeking alternative treatments for depression and anxiety. As research continues, St. John's Wort remains a compelling option for supporting mental health, demonstrating the enduring relevance of herbal medicine in modern therapeutic practices.

Intake:

- 900-1800 mg of standardized extract daily, divided into two or three doses.

Potential Side Effects:

- Photosensitivity, gastrointestinal issues, and potential interactions with medications.

Rhodiola Rosea

Rhodiola Rosea, commonly known as golden root or Arctic root, is a potent adaptogenic herb native to the cold, mountainous regions of Europe and Asia, particularly Siberia. Historically, it has been utilized by Viking warriors to enhance physical strength and endurance, and by Siberian tribes to cope with the harsh climate and stressful conditions. The ancient Greeks also valued Rhodiola, with the Greek physician Dioscorides documenting its medicinal properties as early as the first century AD.

Today, Rhodiola Rosea is celebrated for its ability to combat stress and improve mental resilience. Modern research has shown that Rhodiola can significantly reduce symptoms of fatigue, anxiety, and depression. Its active compounds, rosavin and salidroside, are believed to enhance the body's resistance to physical, chemical, and biological stressors by balancing the release of stress hormones and supporting neurotransmitter function. This makes Rhodiola an effective natural remedy for improving mood, cognitive function, and overall mental well-being.

Currently, Rhodiola Rosea is widely available in supplement form, including capsules, tablets, and teas. It is commonly used by individuals seeking to enhance their energy levels, improve concentration, and reduce stress-related symptoms. As scientific interest in adaptogens grows, Rhodiola Rosea remains a prominent example of how traditional herbal remedies can be integrated into modern health practices to support mental and physical balance.

Intake:

- 200-600 mg of standardized extract daily.

Potential Side Effects:

- Dry mouth, dizziness, and jitteriness.

Valerian Root

Valerian root, derived from the *Valeriana officinalis* plant, is native to Europe and parts of Asia. Its use dates back to ancient Greece and Rome, where it was documented by the physician Hippocrates for its therapeutic properties. In the Middle Ages, it was a popular remedy for various ailments, including insomnia, anxiety, and nervousness. Anglo-Saxon tribes in England revered valerian root for its calming effects, often using it in folk remedies to treat nervous system disorders.

Today, valerian root is widely recognized for its ability to promote relaxation and improve sleep quality. Research suggests that its active compounds, such as valerenic acid and iridoids, interact with gamma-aminobutyric acid (GABA) receptors in the brain, which help to reduce neuronal excitability and induce a calming effect. This makes valerian root a popular natural treatment for insomnia and anxiety, offering an alternative to synthetic sedatives and sleeping pills.

Modern use of valerian root spans various forms, including capsules, tablets, teas, and tinctures. It is frequently employed by individuals seeking to alleviate stress, improve sleep, and enhance overall mental well-being. Scientific studies have validated its effectiveness in reducing sleep latency and improving sleep quality without causing significant side effects, making valerian root a valuable addition to natural health regimens. As interest in herbal medicine continues to grow, valerian root remains a trusted remedy for those looking to achieve a balanced brain and body through natural means.

Intake:

- 400-900 mg of standardized extract, taken 30 minutes to two hours before bedtime.

Potential Side Effects:

- Headaches, dizziness, and gastrointestinal disturbances.

Bacopa Monnieri

Bacopa Monnieri, also known as Brahmi, is an ancient herb native to the wetlands of India, where it has been treasured for its cognitive-enhancing properties for centuries. Its use can be traced back to traditional Ayurvedic medicine, where it was revered as a potent herb for promoting mental clarity, focus, and memory. Brahmi was often prescribed by Ayurvedic practitioners to students and scholars seeking to improve their learning and retention abilities.

Today, Bacopa Monnieri continues to be celebrated for its cognitive benefits and is widely utilized as a natural remedy for enhancing memory and cognitive function. Research suggests that the active compounds in Bacopa, known as bacosides, exhibit neuroprotective effects by reducing oxidative stress, enhancing neurotransmitter activity, and promoting the growth of new nerve cells in the brain. These mechanisms contribute to improved cognitive performance, particularly in areas related to learning, memory, and attention.

Bacopa Monnieri is commonly available in supplement form, including capsules, tablets, and powders. It is frequently incorporated into nootropic stacks and cognitive enhancement formulas to support mental acuity and brain health. As interest in natural approaches to cognitive enhancement grows, Bacopa Monnieri remains a prominent herb in the realm of herbal medicine, offering a gentle yet effective means of optimizing brain function and promoting overall mental well-being.

Intake:

- 300-450 mg of standardized extract daily.

Potential Side Effects:

- Nausea, cramping, and increased bowel movements.

Ginkgo Biloba

Ginkgo Biloba, often referred to as the maidenhair tree, is one of the oldest living tree species on Earth, with a history dating back over 200 million years. Native to China, where it was discovered in the mountains of eastern Asia, Ginkgo Biloba has been revered for its medicinal properties for thousands of years. Ancient Chinese herbalists and Taoist monks prized the tree's fan-shaped leaves for their ability to promote longevity, vitality, and mental clarity. Ginkgo Biloba was traditionally used to support cognitive function, improve circulation, and alleviate respiratory ailments.

Today, Ginkgo Biloba remains a popular herbal remedy for enhancing cognitive function and overall brain health. Research has demonstrated that its active compounds, including flavonoids and terpenoids, possess antioxidant and anti-inflammatory properties that protect neurons from damage, improve blood flow to the brain, and enhance neurotransmitter activity. Studies have shown that Ginkgo Biloba may help improve memory, concentration, and mental performance, making it a valuable supplement for individuals looking to support their cognitive function as they age.

Ginkgo Biloba supplements are widely available in various forms, including capsules, tablets, and extracts. It is frequently used by students, professionals, and older adults seeking to maintain mental acuity and support overall brain health. As scientific interest in herbal medicine continues to grow, Ginkgo Biloba remains a cherished botanical treasure, offering a natural approach to nurturing a balanced brain and body.

Intake:

- 120-240 mg of standardized extract daily.

Potential Side Effects:

- Stomach upset, headache, and allergic skin reactions.

Lemon Balm

Lemon Balm, scientifically known as *Melissa officinalis*, is a fragrant herb belonging to the mint family. Originating from the eastern Mediterranean region, Lemon Balm has a rich history dating back thousands of years. Ancient civilizations, including the Greeks and Romans, revered Lemon Balm for its medicinal properties and soothing aroma. The ancient Greeks believed it to be the "elixir of life" and used it to promote longevity, calm the mind, and improve cognitive function. In medieval Europe, Lemon Balm was cultivated in monastery gardens and used as a remedy for anxiety, insomnia, and digestive issues.

Today, Lemon Balm continues to be valued for its calming and mood-enhancing effects. Research has shown that its active compounds, including rosmarinic acid and citronellal, possess antioxidant and anti-inflammatory properties that help reduce stress, anxiety, and promote relaxation. Lemon Balm is commonly used in herbal teas, tinctures, and supplements to support mental well-being, improve sleep quality, and alleviate symptoms of anxiety and depression.

Lemon Balm's gentle yet effective properties make it a popular choice for individuals seeking natural remedies for stress relief and mood enhancement. As scientific interest in herbal medicine grows, Lemon Balm remains a cherished botanical treasure, offering a soothing and aromatic approach to promoting a balanced brain and body.

Intake:

- 300-600 mg of standardized extract daily.

Potential Side Effects:

- Nausea and allergic reactions.

Lavender

Lavender, scientifically known as *Lavandula angustifolia*, is a versatile herb native to the Mediterranean region, particularly the mountainous areas of northern Africa and the Arabian Peninsula. Its discovery traces back to ancient times, where it was cherished by civilizations such as the ancient Egyptians, Greeks, and Romans. The ancient Egyptians used lavender for its aromatic qualities in perfumes, cosmetics, and embalming rituals. Greeks and Romans, on the other hand, valued lavender for its therapeutic properties, using it to alleviate stress, promote relaxation, and soothe various ailments.

Today, lavender remains a beloved herb with a multitude of uses, particularly in aromatherapy and natural medicine. Research has shown that lavender essential oil contains compounds like linalool and linalyl acetate, which have calming and sedative effects on the nervous system. These properties make lavender a popular choice for reducing anxiety, improving sleep quality, and enhancing overall mental well-being. Lavender is commonly used in essential oil diffusers, bath products, teas, and herbal supplements to promote relaxation and reduce stress levels.

Intake:

- 80-160 mg of lavender oil capsules daily.

Potential Side Effects:

- Nausea, headache, and potential skin irritation.

Passionflower

Passionflower, scientifically known as *Passiflora incarnata*, is a beautiful flowering vine native to the tropical regions of North and South America. Its discovery can be traced back to indigenous tribes of these regions, particularly the Aztecs and Native Americans, who revered it for its calming and sedative properties. The Aztecs used passionflower as a ceremonial herb, believing it to have divine origins and incorporating it into rituals to promote relaxation and induce a state of tranquility. Similarly, Native American tribes utilized passionflower as a remedy for insomnia, anxiety, and nervousness.

Today, passionflower remains a cherished botanical remedy with a wide range of applications in natural medicine. Research has shown that passionflower contains compounds like flavonoids and alkaloids, which exert calming effects on the central nervous system by increasing levels of gamma-aminobutyric acid (GABA), a neurotransmitter that promotes relaxation and reduces neuronal excitability. As a result, passionflower is commonly used to alleviate symptoms of anxiety, improve sleep quality, and enhance overall mental well-being.

Passionflower is available in various forms, including teas, tinctures, capsules, and extracts, and is frequently used as a natural remedy for stress and anxiety. Its gentle yet effective properties make it a popular choice for individuals seeking relaxation and emotional balance.

Intake:

- 400-500 mg of standardized extract daily.

Potential Side Effects:

- Drowsiness, dizziness, and confusion.

Holy Basil (Tulsi)

Holy Basil, scientifically known as *Ocimum sanctum*, is a sacred herb native to the Indian subcontinent, particularly India and Southeast Asia. Its discovery can be traced back to ancient India, where it holds a revered place in Hindu mythology and traditional medicine. Known as "Tulsi" in Sanskrit, Holy Basil is considered a symbol of purity and divine protection, and it is often grown in Hindu households and temples. Ancient Indian scriptures, including the Vedas, mention Holy Basil for its medicinal properties and spiritual significance.

Today, Holy Basil continues to be highly esteemed for its therapeutic benefits and is widely used in Ayurvedic medicine. Research has shown that Holy Basil contains potent antioxidants, such as eugenol and rosmarinic acid, which help reduce inflammation, combat oxidative stress, and support overall health. Holy Basil is renowned for its adaptogenic properties, helping the body adapt to stress and promoting emotional balance. It is commonly used to alleviate symptoms of anxiety, depression, and fatigue, as well as to enhance cognitive function and boost immunity.

Holy Basil is available in various forms, including teas, tinctures, capsules, and essential oils. Its versatility and effectiveness make it a popular choice for individuals seeking natural remedies to support mental and physical well-being. As scientific interest in herbal medicine continues to grow, Holy Basil remains a cherished herb with a long history of promoting a balanced brain and body naturally.

Intake:

- 300-600 mg of standardized extract daily.

Potential Side Effects:

- Mild nausea and potential interactions with blood-thinning medications.

Kava

Kava, scientifically known as *Piper methysticum*, is a plant native to the South Pacific islands, particularly Fiji, Vanuatu, and Tonga. Its discovery can be traced back thousands of years to the indigenous peoples of these regions, where it holds deep cultural and ceremonial significance. In traditional Polynesian societies, kava was revered as a sacred plant used in social gatherings, religious ceremonies, and healing rituals. The drink made from kava roots was believed to induce a sense of relaxation, euphoria, and social bonding.

Today, kava remains an integral part of Pacific Islander culture and is also valued for its potential health benefits. Research has shown that kava contains compounds called kavalactones, which exert calming and sedative effects on the central nervous system by modulating neurotransmitter activity. This makes kava a popular natural remedy for reducing anxiety, promoting relaxation, and improving sleep quality. Kava is commonly consumed as a beverage or used in supplements to support mental well-being and emotional balance.

Despite its long history of traditional use, kava has garnered some controversy due to concerns about potential side effects on the liver. However, when used responsibly and in moderation, kava continues to be embraced by many individuals seeking natural solutions for stress relief and relaxation. As scientific research into its effects continues, kava remains a fascinating botanical.

Intake:

- 100-250 mg of standardized extract, taken two to three times daily.

Potential Side Effects:

- Liver toxicity with long-term use, gastrointestinal discomfort.

Chamomile

Chamomile, derived from the *Matricaria chamomilla* plant, is a daisy-like herb native to Europe and Western Asia. Its discovery can be traced back to ancient Egypt, where it was revered for its medicinal properties and used in various remedies and rituals. Chamomile was considered one of the nine sacred herbs by the Anglo-Saxons and was highly valued for its calming and healing effects. It was commonly used in teas, ointments, and baths to alleviate stress, promote relaxation, and soothe digestive issues.

Today, chamomile remains a beloved herb with a wide range of applications in natural medicine. Research has shown that chamomile contains compounds like apigenin, which exert anti-inflammatory, antioxidant, and sedative effects on the body. This makes chamomile a popular choice for reducing anxiety, improving sleep quality, and soothing gastrointestinal discomfort. Chamomile tea is a common remedy for promoting relaxation and relieving stress, while chamomile supplements are used to support overall mental well-being and digestive health.

As scientific interest in herbal medicine continues to grow, chamomile remains a cherished botanical with a long history of promoting a balanced brain and body naturally. Its gentle yet effective properties make it a popular choice for individuals seeking natural remedies to enhance their well-being and promote emotional balance.

Intake:

  – 200-400 mg of standardized extract daily.

Potential Side Effects:

  – Allergic reactions, particularly in those allergic to ragweed.

Saffron

Saffron, derived from the *Crocus sativus* flower, is a prized spice native to Southwest Asia, particularly Iran, where it has been cultivated for over 3,500 years. Its discovery can be traced back to ancient Mesopotamia, where it was highly valued for its vibrant color, distinct flavor, and medicinal properties. Saffron was used by ancient civilizations, including the Egyptians, Greeks, and Romans, in culinary dishes, perfumes, and traditional medicines.

Throughout history, saffron has held a special place in various cultures and societies. It was considered a symbol of wealth and prestige, often reserved for royalty and used in religious ceremonies and rituals. In traditional Persian medicine, saffron was used to treat a variety of ailments, including depression, anxiety, and insomnia.

Today, saffron continues to be cherished for its unique flavor and potential health benefits. Research has shown that saffron contains compounds like crocin and safranal, which possess antioxidant, anti-inflammatory, and mood-enhancing properties. This makes saffron a popular natural remedy for improving mood, reducing symptoms of depression, and promoting overall mental well-being. Saffron is commonly used in culinary dishes, teas, and supplements to support emotional balance and enhance cognitive function.

Intake:

-   30 mg of standardized extract daily.

Potential Side Effects:

-   Nausea, dizziness, and potential allergic reactions.

Maca Root

Maca root, scientifically known as *Lepidium meyenii*, is a cruciferous vegetable native to the high plateaus of the Andes Mountains in Peru. Its discovery can be traced back over 2,000 years to ancient Incan civilization, where it was highly prized for its energy-boosting properties and revered as a sacred crop. Maca root was consumed by Incan warriors to enhance stamina, strength, and endurance before battle. It was also used by Incan royalty and elite warriors to promote fertility, vitality, and overall well-being.

Throughout history, maca root has maintained its reputation as a powerful adaptogen and nutritional powerhouse. It was traditionally used in Peruvian folk medicine to balance hormones, improve mood, and enhance libido. Today, maca root continues to be valued for its potential health benefits. Research has shown that maca root contains bioactive compounds like macamides and macaenes, which may help regulate hormone levels, reduce stress, and improve sexual function. This makes maca root a popular natural remedy for boosting energy, supporting hormonal balance, and promoting overall mental and physical well-being. Maca root is commonly consumed in powdered form, added to smoothies, beverages, and baked goods, or taken as a supplement.

Intake:

- 1,500-3,000 mg of powdered maca root daily.

Potential Side Effects:

- Gastrointestinal disturbances and increased heart rate in some individuals.

Ginseng

Ginseng, particularly *Panax ginseng* and *Panax quinquefolius*, is a renowned medicinal herb native to East Asia and North America. The discovery of ginseng can be traced back over 5,000 years to ancient China, where it was revered as a powerful tonic for vitality and longevity. It was considered a panacea by Chinese emperors and used extensively in traditional Chinese medicine. Ancient texts, such as the Shennong Ben Cao Jing, document its use in enhancing energy, reducing fatigue, and promoting overall health.

Historically, ginseng was so highly valued that it was often traded for its weight in gold. Native American tribes also discovered the benefits of American ginseng, using it to treat headaches, fever, and digestive issues.

Today, ginseng remains a cornerstone of herbal medicine, widely recognized for its adaptogenic properties. Research indicates that ginseng contains ginsenosides, which have anti-inflammatory, antioxidant, and neuroprotective effects. These compounds help the body cope with stress, enhance cognitive function, and boost energy levels. Modern uses of ginseng include improving mental clarity, reducing anxiety, and supporting immune function.

Ginseng is available in various forms, including teas, extracts, capsules, and powders, making it a versatile supplement for those seeking natural ways to support mental and physical well-being.

Intake:

- 200-400 mg of standardized extract daily.

Potential Side Effects:

- Insomnia, headaches, and digestive issues.

Curcumin

Curcumin, the active compound in turmeric (*Curcuma longa*), is a vibrant yellow spice native to Southeast Asia, particularly India. Its discovery dates back over 4,000 years, with ancient Indian Ayurvedic texts and Chinese medicine praising turmeric for its healing properties. In India, turmeric was not only a culinary staple but also a sacred herb used in religious ceremonies and traditional remedies. Historical records indicate that curcumin was utilized for its anti-inflammatory, antioxidant, and antiseptic properties.

Throughout history, curcumin has maintained its reputation as a powerful medicinal compound. In Ayurvedic and traditional Chinese medicine, turmeric was employed to treat a variety of ailments, including digestive disorders, skin conditions, and joint pain. The golden spice was also a key component in rituals and was believed to purify the body and mind.

Today, curcumin is widely researched for its potential health benefits, particularly its impact on mental and physical well-being. Studies suggest that curcumin's anti-inflammatory and antioxidant properties help protect brain health, reduce symptoms of depression, and enhance cognitive function. It has shown promise in improving mood by modulating neurotransmitters such as serotonin and dopamine.

Curcumin is commonly consumed in the form of turmeric powder, capsules, or extracts. Its versatility and potent health benefits make it a popular supplement for those seeking a balanced approach to well-being.

Intake:

- 500-2,000 mg of standardized extract daily.

Potential Side Effects:

- Gastrointestinal disturbances and potential interactions with medications.

Hops

Hops, derived from the *Humulus lupulus* plant, are best known for their role in brewing beer, but they also have a rich history as a medicinal herb. Native to Europe, Western Asia, and North America, hops have been used for centuries for their calming and health-promoting properties. The discovery of hops as a brewing ingredient dates back to the early Middle Ages, around the 9th century, in regions that are now Germany. Monastic communities were instrumental in cultivating and utilizing hops not only for brewing but also for medicinal purposes.

Historically, hops were used by various cultures to treat ailments such as anxiety, insomnia, and digestive issues. For example, in ancient Europe, hop-filled pillows were used to promote restful sleep. The sedative properties of hops made them a valuable remedy for those suffering from restlessness and anxiety.

Today, hops continue to be recognized for their health benefits beyond brewing. They contain compounds such as xanthohumol and humulone, which have anti-inflammatory, antioxidant, and neuroprotective effects. These properties make hops a popular natural remedy for supporting mental health, particularly in reducing anxiety and improving sleep quality. Hops are also used to support digestive health, thanks to their bitter principles that stimulate appetite and aid digestion.

Modern research has validated many of these traditional uses, highlighting hops' potential in promoting relaxation, reducing stress, and supporting overall well-being.

Intake:

- 300-500 mg of standardized extract daily.

Potential Side Effects:

- Drowsiness and digestive issues.

Skullcap

Skullcap, derived from the *Scutellaria* genus of flowering plants, has a long history of use in traditional medicine, particularly in North America and Asia. Native to these regions, skullcap was discovered by indigenous tribes and used extensively for its calming and healing properties. In North America, Native American tribes utilized American skullcap (*Scutellaria lateriflora*) as a remedy for anxiety, insomnia, and convulsions. It was often brewed into teas or made into tinctures to treat various ailments and to promote relaxation.

In Asia, particularly in China, Chinese skullcap (*Scutellaria baicalensis*) has been used for over 2,000 years in traditional Chinese medicine. Known as "Huang Qin," it was employed to treat inflammation, infections, and respiratory conditions. The root of Chinese skullcap was a crucial component in many herbal formulations aimed at balancing the body's internal energies and supporting overall health.

Today, skullcap continues to be valued for its health benefits. It contains bioactive compounds such as flavonoids, baicalin, and wogonin, which have anti-inflammatory, antioxidant, and neuroprotective effects. These properties make skullcap an effective natural remedy for reducing anxiety, improving sleep quality, and protecting against neurological disorders. Skullcap is also used to support cardiovascular health and to combat oxidative stress, contributing to overall well-being.

Intake:

- 300-600 mg of standardized extract daily.

Potential Side Effects:

- Drowsiness, confusion, and potential liver damage with long-term use.

Gotu Kola

Gotu Kola, scientifically known as *Centella asiatica*, is a perennial herb native to the wetlands of Asia, including India, China, Indonesia, and Sri Lanka. Its discovery dates back thousands of years, where it was prominently featured in ancient Ayurvedic and traditional Chinese medicine. In India, Gotu Kola is often referred to as "Brahmi," named after the Hindu god Brahma, symbolizing its revered status. The herb was used by yogis and monks to enhance meditation practices due to its believed effects on mental clarity and tranquility.

In traditional medicine, Gotu Kola has been used to treat a wide range of ailments. Ancient Chinese texts describe its use in promoting longevity and enhancing mental function. Legend has it that the renowned Chinese herbalist Li Ching-Yuen, who allegedly lived over 200 years, attributed his long life to daily consumption of Gotu Kola.

Modern research has validated many of Gotu Kola's traditional uses. The herb contains bioactive compounds such as triterpenoids, which have been shown to possess anti-inflammatory, antioxidant, and neuroprotective properties. These compounds help in enhancing cognitive function, reducing anxiety, and promoting overall mental well-being. Gotu Kola is also known for its ability to improve circulation, support wound healing, and maintain skin health.

Today, Gotu Kola is used globally as a natural supplement to support brain health, reduce stress, and improve memory and cognitive function.

Intake:

- 500-1,000 mg of standardized extract daily.

Potential Side Effects:

- Stomach upset, headaches, and dizziness.

Mucuna Pruriens

Mucuna Pruriens, commonly known as velvet bean, is a tropical legume native to Africa and tropical Asia. Its discovery and use date back thousands of years in Ayurvedic medicine, where it is known as "Kapikachhu." Traditionally, it was used to support overall vitality, enhance mood, and improve neurological health. In India, ancient texts such as the Charaka Samhita and Sushruta Samhita detail its applications in treating nervous disorders, aphrodisiac purposes, and enhancing sexual health.

The seeds of *Mucuna Pruriens* are particularly notable for their high content of L-DOPA, a precursor to the neurotransmitter dopamine. Dopamine plays a critical role in regulating mood, motivation, and movement. Historically, velvet bean was also used by African and Caribbean communities to treat conditions such as snake bites and to improve male fertility. The beans were often roasted and ground into a powder, which was then consumed in various forms.

Modern research has shed light on the numerous health benefits of Mucuna Pruriens. Its neuroprotective and antioxidant properties help protect brain cells from damage, potentially aiding in the management of neurodegenerative diseases such as Parkinson's. Additionally, its mood-enhancing effects can alleviate symptoms of depression and anxiety by boosting dopamine levels.

Intake:

- 200-500 mg of standardized extract daily.

Potential Side Effects:

- Nausea, vomiting, and potential interactions with medications.

Relative Strength of Herbal supplements

Herbal supplements vary greatly in their strength and benefits, each offering unique impacts on your mental health. This visual presentation illustrates the relative potency of various herbal supplements in supporting mental well-being, based on scientific evidence. The bar chart categorizes each supplement on a scale of 1 to 10. Supplements such as Ashwagandha and St. John's Wort are rated highly, indicating strong benefits for mental health, while others like Maca Root and Hops are noted for their moderate impact. Let this chart aid you in quickly identifying the most effective herbal options for your mental well-being.

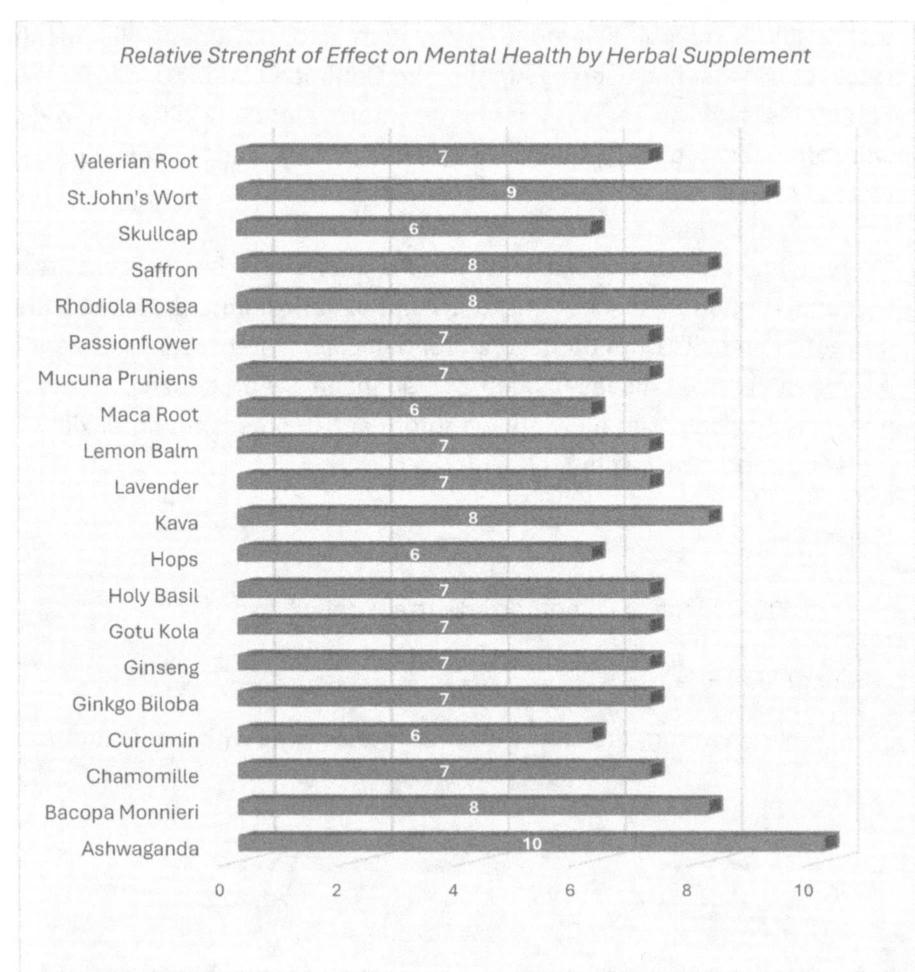

Essential Guidelines for Herbal Supplementation

Incorporating herbal supplements into your routine can provide significant benefits for your emotional and overall health. However, it's essential to consult with a healthcare professional before starting any new supplement regimen, especially if you have existing health conditions or are taking other medications. By understanding the effects, proper dosages, and potential side effects of these herbal supplements, you can make informed decisions to support your mental well-being effectively. Never take a higher dose than written on the supplement's dosage information and always follow the guidelines. Additionally, please note that the dosages mentioned in this book may deviate from the prescribed dosage on the supplement bottle.

Nootropics

In your journey to enhance mental well-being, you may encounter the term "nootropics"—a class of substances known for their cognitive-enhancing properties. Nootropics vary greatly in their strength and benefits, each offering unique impacts on mental health. Whether you're looking to boost memory, improve focus, or elevate creativity, understanding nootropics can be a powerful tool in your mental wellness toolkit.

What Are Nootropics?

Nootropics, often referred to as "smart drugs," are substances that may improve memory, enhance cognition, support motivation, and drive creative capacity. This term, coined in the 1970s by Romanian psychologist Corneliu E. Giurgea, originally described substances that activate certain brain functions, particularly among those with impaired functioning. Today, nootropics encompass a broad range of natural and synthetic substances that can impact cognitive function.

Nootropics fall into two primary categories:

Dietary Supplements: Made from herbs, vitamins, minerals, and other natural compounds, these nootropics are often marketed as proprietary blends. Their efficacy can be challenging to substantiate, as they are not regulated by the FDA like medications.

Pharmaceuticals: This category includes prescription medications like Ritalin and Adderall, which are regulated by the FDA.

Effectiveness

Nootropics can enhance memory, reduce brain fog, boost mood, and improve mental clarity. However, their effectiveness varies. Some nootropics have well-documented benefits, while others rely more on anecdotal evidence. More research is needed, especially on healthy individuals, to fully understand the long-term safety and effectiveness of many nootropics.

Benefits of Nootropics

The potential benefits of nootropics include:

- Enhanced memory and learning ability

- Improved focus and attention span

- Increased motivation and mood

- Enhanced creativity

- Neuroprotection and improved brain health

Risks of Nootropics

Despite their potential benefits, nootropics carry risks, including:

- Side effects ranging from mild (headaches) to severe (cardiovascular issues)

- Risk of dependency or addiction

- Potential drug interactions

- Certain unknown long-term effects

For example, prescription nootropics for ADHD, such as Adderall or Ritalin, can be misused and have side effects like insomnia and increased blood pressure. Dietary supplements, being less regulated, might contain undisclosed or unsafe ingredients. It's crucial to never take a higher dose than written on the supplement's dosage information and always follow the guidelines. Also, note that dosages mentioned in this book deviate from the prescribed dosage on supplement bottles.

Nootropics, also known as "smart drugs," offer the potential to unlock your brain's latent abilities, enhancing cognition, creativity, and motivation. They work through various mechanisms, such as enhancing neurotransmitter levels, improving blood flow to the brain, or protecting against neuronal damage. As you explore these compounds, particularly pharmaceuticals, remember to approach their use with caution and awareness. The next section of this chapter will explore the specifics of popular nootropics, guiding you to make informed choices for your mental and overall health.

Alpha-GPC (L-Alpha glycerylphosphorylcholine)

Alpha-GPC (alpha-glycerophosphocholine or choline alphoscerate) is a choline-containing phospholipid notable for its rapid absorption and ability to cross the blood-brain barrier. Once ingested, it metabolizes into choline and glycerol-1-phosphate. Choline, a precursor of acetylcholine, plays a vital role in memory, attention, and cognitive function.

Alpha-GPC is primarily explored for its cognitive-enhancement properties. While rodent studies show improvements in learning and memory, such benefits in healthy humans are yet to be confirmed. However, in older adults with mild to moderate dementia, alpha-GPC has demonstrated improvements in cognitive symptoms such as memory and attention impairment. Additionally, it may enhance the effectiveness of acetylcholinesterase inhibitors used in Alzheimer's treatment, potentially improving both behavioral and cognitive outcomes. A 2022 study indicated that alpha-GPC might benefit glioblastoma patients when combined with conventional treatments, showcasing its potential broader neuroprotective effects.

Despite its benefits, recent concerns highlight alpha-GPC's potential link to cardiovascular disease due to its role in synthesizing trimethylamine-N-oxide (TMAO). A 2021 cohort study suggested a possible increased risk of stroke with long-term use, though further research is needed to confirm these findings.

Alpha-GPC works by enhancing acetylcholine synthesis in the brain, which is crucial for memory, motivation, arousal, and attention. Known by several names, including alpha-glycerylphosphorylcholine and choline alphoscerate, alpha-GPC continues to be a subject of interest for its potential to enhance cognitive function and support mental health.

N-Acetylcysteine (NAC)

N-acetylcysteine (NAC) is a stable, acetylated form of the amino acid L-cysteine, renowned for its antioxidant and anti-inflammatory properties. NAC effectively crosses the blood-brain barrier, increasing levels of the powerful antioxidant glutathione, which is rapidly depleted by stress, disease, and drug toxicity. This elevation in glutathione levels is crucial for brain health, protecting neurons from oxidative damage and reducing inflammation.

Research highlights NAC's potential in alleviating symptoms of various mental health disorders. Its ability to modulate glutamate and dopamine neurotransmission shows promise for treating conditions like schizophrenia and substance use disorder. Additionally, NAC has been found to reduce proinflammatory cytokines, which are often elevated in individuals with depression and anxiety. By lowering these cytokines, NAC can help mitigate inflammation-related mental health issues.

The cytoprotective effects of NAC further support cognitive function and mental clarity. By enhancing glutathione production, NAC safeguards against neuronal damage, potentially improving mood, motivation, and overall cognitive performance. Although more research is needed to fully understand its impact, NAC's ability to boost antioxidant levels and modulate neurotransmission positions it as a valuable supplement for mental well-being. With its proven safety and effectiveness, NAC offers a promising approach to enhancing mental health and cognitive function.

L-Theanine

L-theanine, a naturally occurring amino acid found in tea, offers significant benefits for mental health. Unlike standard amino acids, L-theanine isn't used in protein synthesis but is renowned for its stress and anxiety-reducing properties. Supplementing with L-theanine can help alleviate stress and anxiety, particularly in acutely stressful situations. It has also been shown to prevent stress-induced increases in blood pressure. Studies suggest that L-theanine can lower depression and anxiety scores in both healthy individuals and those with major depressive disorder.

Additionally, L-theanine may enhance cognitive function, including attention, executive function, and memory. However, it can impair executive function and attentional control during emotionally charged or stressful mental tasks. Moreover, L-theanine promotes a relaxed state in the brain by increasing alpha-wave activity, which is associated with relaxation and stress reduction.

L-theanine also shows promise in improving sleep quality by fostering relaxation. While most evidence comes from studies on healthy individuals, L-theanine's ability to reduce stress and anxiety and improve sleep and cognitive function makes it a valuable supplement for mental well-being. More research is needed to confirm these effects in individuals with chronic conditions, but L-theanine's neuroprotective and anxiety-reducing properties are well-documented.

Ginkgo Biloba

Ginkgo biloba, derived from the leaves of the ginkgo tree, is a popular supplement for enhancing mental well-being. These leaves contain various bioactive compounds, such as flavonoids and terpenoids, which contribute to its potential cognitive benefits. Ginkgo biloba is particularly noted for its ability to improve cognitive function in individuals with dementia. Preliminary evidence also suggests that it can enhance cognitive performance in healthy middle-aged and older adults, though its effects on younger individuals remain inconclusive.

One of the primary benefits of Ginkgo biloba is its potential to support mental clarity and memory. It may work by improving blood flow to the brain, reducing oxidative stress, and inhibiting the neurotoxic effects of amyloid beta, although the exact mechanisms are not fully understood.

Ginkgo biloba is generally considered safe, with no significant safety concerns identified in clinical trials. While there have been isolated reports of increased bleeding risk and seizures in individuals with epilepsy, a meta-analysis of 18 randomized controlled trials found no higher risk of bleeding in those taking standardized extracts. However, rare cases of seizures and potential carcinogenic effects in rodent studies highlight the need for cautious use. Overall, Ginkgo biloba holds promise for enhancing mental health, particularly in older adults and those with cognitive impairments.

Lion's Mane Mushroom

Lion's mane (*Hericium erinaceus*) is a mushroom recognized for its potential mental health benefits, particularly its neuroprotective and antioxidant properties. It has been used in traditional Chinese medicine for centuries. The mushroom contains bioactive compounds, including polysaccharides and terpenoids, which contribute to its effects on cognitive function and mental health.

Several studies have explored Lion's mane's impact on cognitive decline and neurodegenerative conditions. In one randomized controlled trial (RCT), individuals with mild Alzheimer's disease showed improved scores in the Instrumental Activities of Daily Living (IADL) test after taking Lion's mane for 49 weeks, although other cognitive tests showed no significant differences. Another study demonstrated that 3 grams of Lion's mane powder daily improved cognitive function in individuals with mild cognitive decline, but the benefits diminished after stopping the supplement. An RCT with healthy older adults also showed improved Mini-Mental State Examination (MMSE) scores, indicating potential for preventing cognitive decline.

Lion's mane may also reduce anxiety and depression symptoms. Studies involving menopausal women and overweight individuals reported improvements in mental health after supplementation. These findings suggest that Lion's mane could support cognitive function and mental well-being, but more research is needed to confirm these effects in broader populations.

Creatine

Creatine, a molecule produced from amino acids such as arginine, glycine, and methionine, is essential for energy production in the body. Primarily synthesized in the liver, kidneys, and pancreas, it stores high-energy phosphate groups in the form of phosphocreatine, which helps regenerate ATP, the primary energy carrier, especially during intense physical or mental activities. While it is commonly associated with physical performance, creatine has notable mental health benefits as well.

Research indicates that creatine supplementation can reduce mental fatigue in stressful situations, such as sleep deprivation or exhaustive exercise. It may also enhance memory, particularly in individuals with low creatine levels, including vegetarians and older adults. Preliminary studies suggest that creatine could alleviate symptoms of depression in individuals with major depressive disorder or bipolar disorder. This is potentially due to its role in maintaining energy homeostasis in brain cells, which may help stabilize mood and cognitive functions.

The pro-energetic properties of creatine extend to the central nervous system, promoting energy availability and supporting brain health. Although more research is needed to fully understand its impact on cognitive performance and mental health, current findings highlight creatine's potential as a beneficial supplement for improving mental well-being and cognitive resilience.

Acetyl-L-Carnitine (ALCAR)

L-carnitine, a compound derived from the amino acids lysine and methionine, plays a crucial role in energy production by transporting long-chain fatty acids into mitochondria. Its acetylated form, acetyl-L-carnitine (ALCAR), is notable for crossing the blood-brain barrier more efficiently, making it particularly relevant for mental health. Research suggests that L-carnitine and ALCAR may benefit cognitive function and mental health. ALCAR, in particular, has shown potential in improving symptoms of depression and cognitive decline. Studies have demonstrated that ALCAR supplementation can enhance memory and cognitive performance, particularly in older adults and individuals with mild cognitive impairment.

The neuroprotective effects of L-carnitine are attributed to its antioxidant properties, which protect brain cells from oxidative stress and inflammation. Additionally, L-carnitine has been observed to increase levels of nitric oxide, which improves blood flow and may further support brain health. In individuals with major depressive disorder or bipolar disorder, preliminary evidence suggests that L-carnitine supplementation can alleviate depressive symptoms, although more research is needed to confirm these findings.

Animal studies have also highlighted L-carnitine's potential to restore levels of neurotransmitters such as serotonin, norepinephrine, and dopamine, which are often depleted in stress-related conditions. This mechanism may explain its antidepressant-like effects observed in experimental settings. Overall, while L-carnitine is widely recognized for its role in physical performance, its potential mental health benefits, including cognitive enhancement and mood improvement, are gaining increasing attention, warranting further investigation.

Phenylpiracetam

Phenylpiracetam, a nootropic in the racetam family and a phenyl derivative of piracetam, has significant effects on mental health. It is reported to be more neuroprotective than piracetam and also has psychostimulatory properties that enhance physical performance. Research indicates that phenylpiracetam is effective in mitigating cognitive decline, particularly in conditions like dementia and stroke, where it is used for over a month. However, its benefits for cognitive decline from traumatic brain injury are less clear.

Studies have shown that phenylpiracetam can reduce the rate and severity of cognitive decline. One notable study in rats highlighted that the R-isomer of phenylpiracetam significantly improved cognitive functions in healthy young rats, although the racemic mixture, which is commonly sold, did not outperform the control group. This suggests that while phenylpiracetam may enhance cognition in youth, its psychostimulatory properties, observed with both the racemic mixture and the R-isomer, are distinct.

Phenylpiracetam's ability to protect neurons and its potential to improve cognitive performance make it a promising supplement for mental health. It works by enhancing neurotransmitter activity, increasing brain blood flow, and providing neuroprotection. These mechanisms help reduce mental fatigue, improve focus, and enhance overall cognitive function. The psychostimulatory effects also contribute to increased alertness and mental energy, making it beneficial for individuals needing cognitive enhancement and mental clarity.

Despite these promising effects, the optimal dosage of phenylpiracetam is not yet well-established, and its long-term safety and efficacy require further research. Nevertheless, its potential to support mental health through cognitive enhancement and neuroprotection positions phenylpiracetam as a noteworthy nootropic.

Noopept

Noopept, or N-phenylacetyl-L-prolylglycine ethyl ester, is a synthetic pharmaceutical created by a Russian company, classified as a nootropic due to its neuroprotective and cognitive-enhancing properties. Its structure is based on piracetam, another well-known nootropic. Preliminary research indicates that Noopept may benefit brain health, primarily through studies on rodents with brain damage caused by toxins or oxygen deprivation. These studies suggest that Noopept can enhance cognitive functions and protect neural structures.

In one of the few human trials, Noopept supplementation improved cognitive function in a small group of individuals with mild cognitive impairment (MCI) resulting from a stroke. However, these findings are not yet independently replicated, warranting cautious optimism about its efficacy.

The potential mental health benefits of Noopept include increased levels of brain-derived neurotrophic factor (BDNF), a protein crucial for establishing neural connections and neurotransmission. Noopept may also interact with neurotransmitter receptors involved in learning and cognitive function, such as glutamatergic and cholinergic receptors. These interactions could underlie its cognitive-enhancing effects.

However, Noopept's safety profile requires more research. Reported side effects include sleep disturbances, irritability, increased blood pressure, dizziness, headaches, and gastrointestinal symptoms. There is limited data on the long-term effects of Noopept, and its safety remains uncertain.

Despite its potential, Noopept's efficacy and safety in improving mental health need more rigorous and extensive research to confirm its benefits and understand its mechanisms fully. For supplementation, the suggested dose ranges from 10 to 30 mg daily for up to 56 days, but optimal dosing for humans is yet to be determined.

Aniracetam

Aniracetam, a compound within the racetam family, is recognized for its potential mental health benefits. Structurally a pyrrolidone, Aniracetam is fat-soluble and should be ingested with fatty acids. It is also cholinergic, meaning it influences the neurotransmitter acetylcholine, which plays a critical role in learning and memory.

Aniracetam acts as a positive modulator of AMPA receptors, which are excitatory receptors in the brain. This modulation leads to a controlled and prolonged neurological stimulation by decreasing the rate of receptor desensitization. Given that AMPA receptors vary in structure across different brain regions, Aniracetam's effects can differ depending on the brain area it influences. This unique interaction is linked to improved cognitive processes, such as 'collective and holistic thinking' or the ability to integrate various pieces of information. Additionally, Aniracetam increases blood flow and activity in the association cortex, the brain area involved in complex cognitive functions.

Currently, Aniracetam is under study for its potential to alleviate symptoms of depression and other central nervous system (CNS) disorders, including Alzheimer's disease. Its modulation of AMPA receptors suggests it might help manage these conditions by enhancing synaptic plasticity and neuronal communication.

Sulbutiamine

Sulbutiamine is a synthetic derivative of thiamine (vitamin B1) known for its potential cognitive and mental health benefits. Structurally designed to enhance thiamine's efficacy, it easily crosses the blood-brain barrier, making it more effective in the central nervous system. One of its primary mental health benefits is its potential to improve mood and reduce fatigue. Studies suggest that sulbutiamine can alleviate symptoms of asthenia, a condition characterized by chronic fatigue, which is often linked to depression and anxiety.

Additionally, sulbutiamine may enhance memory and cognitive function. It has been observed to improve both short-term and long-term memory, likely due to its influence on cholinergic and dopaminergic neurotransmission. This makes it a promising supplement for individuals experiencing cognitive decline or those who need to boost their cognitive performance under stress.

Another notable effect of sulbutiamine is its potential role in treating mild cognitive impairment and early stages of Alzheimer's disease. Preliminary studies indicate that it can enhance attention and memory, providing a cognitive boost for individuals with these conditions. However, more extensive research is needed to confirm these findings and establish its efficacy.

Despite its promising effects, sulbutiamine's optimal dosage and regimen are not well-defined. Human studies typically use a daily dose of 400 mg, but the ideal dosage, including whether it should be taken with meals or in divided doses, remains unclear. Overall, sulbutiamine appears to be a beneficial supplement for improving mood, reducing fatigue, and enhancing cognitive functions, although further research is essential to fully understand its potential and optimize its use.

Huperzine A

Huperzine-A, a compound derived from Huperziceae herbs, is known for its significant mental health benefits. As an acetylcholinesterase inhibitor, it prevents the breakdown of acetylcholine, a neurotransmitter crucial for learning and memory. This leads to increased levels of acetylcholine in the brain, enhancing cognitive functions and promoting better mental performance.

One of the primary benefits of Huperzine-A is its potential to improve memory and learning. By maintaining higher levels of acetylcholine, it supports cognitive processes and has shown promise in preliminary trials for treating Alzheimer's disease. Its neuroprotective properties may help slow the progression of this neurodegenerative condition, offering hope for those affected by memory loss and cognitive decline.

Huperzine-A is also valued for its ability to enhance focus and mental clarity. This makes it a popular supplement among students and professionals who require sustained mental effort and concentration. Additionally, it may help reduce cognitive fatigue, making it easier to stay mentally sharp during prolonged periods of study or work.

Studies have indicated that Huperzine-A is a relatively safe compound, with no significant side effects observed at typical supplementation doses. It is usually taken in doses ranging from 50 to 200 mcg daily, and its long half-life of 10-14 hours allows for flexible dosing schedules. Many users opt for cycling their supplementation, taking Huperzine-A for 2-4 weeks followed by a break to maintain its effectiveness.

Overall, Huperzine-A offers a promising natural approach to boosting cognitive function, improving memory, and supporting mental health, particularly in the context of age-related cognitive decline and high cognitive demands.

Phosphatidylserine

Phosphatidylserine (PS) is a crucial phospholipid in the brain, constituting 15% of its total phospholipids and playing a significant role in mental health. Originally derived from cattle brains, PS is now primarily sourced from soy due to safety concerns. It is often studied in conjunction with omega-3 fatty acids like DHA and EPA, as PS is linked to DHA in the brain, enhancing its cognitive functions.

PS supplementation has shown promise in improving cognitive functions, particularly in adults over 50. Several randomized controlled trials have indicated that daily doses of 100-300 mg for 2-6 months can enhance memory and cognitive performance, although more research is needed to confirm these benefits. Additionally, PS may help reduce perceived stress levels in individuals with chronic stress by modulating the hypothalamus-pituitary-adrenal (HPA) axis, which regulates the body's stress response. By potentially lowering levels of ACTH and cortisol, PS can contribute to stress reduction and improved mental clarity.

In terms of safety, PS appears to be well-tolerated. Studies have reported minimal adverse effects, with gastrointestinal discomfort being the most common side effect, which can be mitigated by taking PS with food. This suggests that PS is a relatively safe option for those seeking to enhance cognitive function and manage stress.

PS also supports communication between neurons by crossing the blood-brain barrier, impacting memory, learning, and language processes. This makes it a valuable supplement for both age-related cognitive decline and general mental health maintenance. Overall, phosphatidylserine holds significant potential for improving mental health by enhancing cognitive functions and reducing stress.

Centrophenoxine

Centrophenoxine, marketed under the brand name Lucidril, is a cholinergic compound known for its potential mental health benefits. It contains Dimethylaminoethanol (DMAE), which is more effectively transported to the brain when taken as Centrophenoxine. This compound is readily available over the counter or online.

Centrophenoxine is recognized for its neuroprotective and cognitive-enhancing properties. It is particularly effective in reversing signs of aging in the brain, such as the accumulation of waste products, when taken in high doses over a short period. In addition to its anti-aging effects, Centrophenoxine can be used continuously at lower doses to enhance overall neural function and protect brain health.

Studies suggest that Centrophenoxine improves cognitive function by increasing acetylcholine levels, a neurotransmitter crucial for learning and memory. This enhancement in acetylcholine can lead to better memory retention, faster recall, and improved mental clarity. Moreover, Centrophenoxine's antioxidant properties help reduce oxidative stress in the brain, which is beneficial for maintaining cognitive health and potentially slowing the progression of neurodegenerative diseases.

For younger individuals seeking cognitive enhancement and neuroprotection, a typical dosage is 250 mg taken one to three times daily. In contrast, older adults aiming to reduce brain waste products and combat age-related cognitive decline might take three to six doses of 250 mg daily.

Overall, Centrophenoxine offers significant potential for improving mental health by boosting cognitive function, protecting neurons, and mitigating age-related brain deterioration. Its accessibility and effectiveness make it a valuable supplement for those looking to enhance their mental acuity and preserve brain health.

5-HTP

5-HTP, a precursor to serotonin, holds significant implications for mental health. Serotonin, known as the "happiness neurotransmitter," influences mood regulation, sleep patterns, appetite, and emotional stability. By increasing serotonin levels in the brain's neurons, 5-HTP supplementation is believed to potentially alleviate symptoms of depression, although the evidence remains mixed and inconclusive. Some studies suggest that 5-HTP may reduce depression symptoms when taken alone or alongside standard treatments like SSRIs, comparable in effectiveness to certain antidepressant medications over short periods.

Beyond depression, 5-HTP has been explored for its role in appetite control, with observations of reduced calorie intake and increased satiety in overweight individuals. However, its impact on conditions like migraine prevention, tension headaches, fibromyalgia, and Parkinson's disease remains uncertain due to conflicting research outcomes.

While 5-HTP offers potential mental health benefits, it is not without drawbacks. Common side effects include nausea, abdominal discomfort, and diarrhea, with less frequent reports of insomnia, fatigue, and headaches. In rare cases, high doses have been linked to serotonin syndrome, a serious condition characterized by excessively high serotonin levels.

In conclusion, while 5-HTP shows promise in augmenting serotonin levels and potentially aiding mental well-being, its clinical benefits and safety profile necessitate further rigorous investigation. Understanding its nuanced effects on mood, sleep, and overall mental health remains pivotal in shaping its therapeutic applications effectively.

SAM-e

S-adenosylmethionine (SAMe), a naturally occurring compound in the body, plays a crucial role in mental health by serving as a methyl donor in various biochemical reactions. In conditions like depression and osteoarthritis, lower levels of SAMe have been observed, suggesting a therapeutic potential. Clinical studies indicate that daily supplementation with SAMe at doses ranging from 800mg to 1600mg can be as effective as certain pharmaceutical treatments for alleviating symptoms of both depression and osteoarthritis, with noticeable improvements often seen within a few weeks of consistent use.

SAMe operates within a regulated range in the bloodstream, influencing metabolic processes critical for maintaining health. While generally well-tolerated, SAMe supplementation may lead to rare instances of manic episodes, particularly in individuals without a history of bipolar disorder. This phenomenon underscores the importance of monitoring its effects, despite the absence of clear pathological links to such reactions.

In the context of diabetes, SAMe's impact on glucose control remains less established compared to its effects on mood and joint health. Nonetheless, its role as a methyl donor suggests broader implications for metabolic support and potential therapeutic applications in conditions characterized by SAMe deficiency.

Overall, SAMe emerges as a promising adjunct therapy for managing depression and osteoarthritis, offering a natural alternative with fewer reported side effects compared to conventional treatments. Continued research is essential to elucidate its precise mechanisms and optimize therapeutic strategies for maximizing its benefits in mental health and beyond.

Dosage

Alpha-GPC	For attenuating symptoms of cognitive decline, almost all studies used a dosage of 1,200 mg per day, divided into three doses of 400 mg. For boosting power output, studies have used a dosage of 300–600 mg, supplemented 30–60 minutes prior to exercise.
N-Acetylcysteine (NAC)	Orally, NAC is most often given in the dosage range of 600–1,800 mg daily (often divided into two or three daily doses), although higher doses are sometimes used in clinical research.
L-Theanine	Clinical studies typically use L-theanine at a dosage of 100–400 milligrams (mg) per day
Ginkgo Biloba	For cognitive enhancement, take 120-240mg, one to four hours before performance. To alleviate cognitive decline in older adults, take 40-120mg, three times a day.
Lion's Mane Mushroom	Clinical studies investigating lion's mane mushroom have utilized dosages ranging from 1050–3000 mg, divided into three to four daily doses. Nevertheless, the optimal dose remains uncertain, and the minimum effective concentration may vary depending on the specific target system.
Creatine	In most studies, supplementation involved an initial loading protocol of around 0.3 grams per kilogram of bodyweight per day (typically divided into four equal doses throughout the day) for 5–7 days followed by a daily maintenance dose of at least 0.03 g/kg of bodyweight. For a 180 lb (82 kg) person, this translates to a loading dose of 25 g/day and a maintenance dose of at least 2.5 g/day. The "alternative" to creatine loading involves simply taking a smaller dose (usually 3–5 g) of creatine every day.
Acetyl-L-Carnitine (ALCAR)	The standard dose for L-carnitine is between 500–2000 milligrams per day (mg/day). Supplementation with up to 2000 mg/day of L-carnitine is considered safe for humans. There are various other forms of carnitine supplementation available: The equivalent dosage is up to about 2700 mg/day for acetyl-L-carnitine and up to about 2900 mg/day for propionyl L-carnitine.
Phenylpiracetam	Phenylpiracetam is taken at a dosage of 100-200mg acutely, and this dose is taken 2-3 times per day (totalling a daily range of 200-600mg). The lower range seems effective, but the optimal dosage is not yet known.
Noopept	To supplement Noopept, take 10 – 30 mg, once a day, for up to 56 days at a time. More research is needed to determine the optimal human dose for Noopept.

Aniracetam	Doses between 10 mg/kg bodyweight and 100 mg/kg bodyweight have been used in rats with efficacy in laboratory settings. Limited human evidence finds that oral doses in the 1,000-1,500 mg range (over the course of a day) tend to be effective. Doses as low as 400 mg have been reported to have some efficacy, and it is common to take the above 1,000-1,500 mg aniracetam in two divided doses of 500-750 mg twice daily with meals.
Sulbutiamine	Human studies using sulbutiamine supplementation have used 400mg daily. It is not clear if this is near the optimal dosage, and an ideal dosing regimen (with or without meals and how many divided doses a day) is not currently known.
Huperzine A	Supplementation of huperzine-A tends to be in the range of 50-200mcg daily, and while this can be divided into multiple dosages throughout the day it tends to be taken at a single dose. Supplementation of huperzine-A does not require food to be coingested with it and can be taken in a fasted state.
Phosphatidylserine	A standard dosage of phosphatidylserine (PS) is 300 mg daily, divided into 3 doses of 100 mg each. This dosage seems to be effective as a daily preventative against cognitive decline, and 100 mg once daily may provide some degree of benefit (but might be less beneficial than 300 mg). Studies in children and adolescents for the purpose of attention improvement tend to use 200 mg, and a dose of 200–400 mg has been used in adult non-elderly humans with success. Animal evidence tends to use a dose correlating to 550mg as well.
Centrophenoxine	For therapeutic usage in reducing lipofuscin (for the aged) 3-6 doses of 250mg centrophenoxine is generally touted. For younger individuals seeking neurological enhancement and neuronal protection, 1-3 doses of 250mg suffices.
5-HTP	5-HTP is usually taken orally in capsule form. It can be taken once daily or in divided doses (i.e., the total daily dose is split into two or three doses). For depression, most studies have used dosages in the range of 200 mg to 300 mg daily for up to 1 year. For weight loss or appetite regulation, 5-HTP has been used in the range of 750 mg to 900 mg daily for up to 6 weeks.
SAM-e	Supplementation of S-adenosylmethionine tends to be in the 600-1,200mg range over the course of a day, divided into two or three separated doses with meals. The higher dosage (1,200mg) tends to be used more often, with the lower dosage (600mg) being used to cut costs.

Nootropics offer a range of benefits for mental and overall health by enhancing cognitive function, reducing stress, and supporting cellular health. However, it is crucial to consult with a healthcare professional before starting any new supplement regimen to ensure safety and efficacy. Understanding the effects, proper dosages, and potential side effects of these nootropics can help you make informed decisions to support your mental well-being effectively.

Relative Strength of Effect on Mental Health by Nootropic

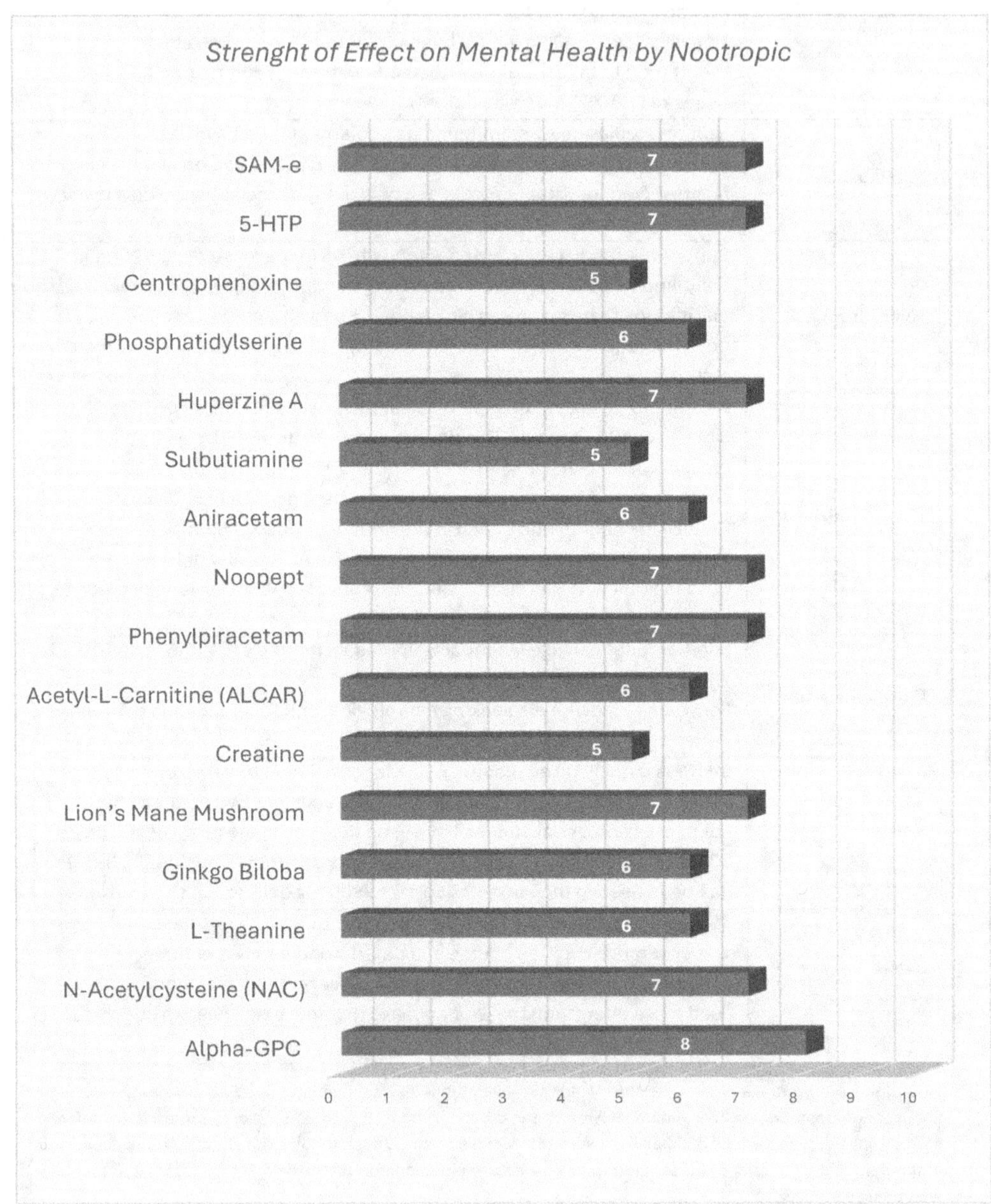

Which Nutrition to Avoid?

This chapter is a pivotal guide in your journey towards achieving optimal mental and physical well-being. While much emphasis is often placed on the nutrients and supplements that can enhance our mental health, it is equally crucial to understand which elements of our diet can hinder our progress.

Maintaining a balanced diet is essential not only for physical health but also for mental clarity and emotional stability. However, certain foods and substances can have detrimental effects, often undermining our efforts to stay healthy. This chapter will explore ten specific nutritional elements that should be avoided or limited, because they have the most negative impact on your mental state. By understanding their adverse impacts on both mental and overall health, you can make more informed choices about what to include and exclude from your diet.

We will explore why these elements should be limited, outlining their potential side effects and offering maximum intake guidelines to help you navigate your dietary choices. This knowledge will empower you to protect your mental health by avoiding substances that can cause harm, thus maintaining a healthy body as the foundation of a healthy brain.

Stay motivated and curious as you uncover the content of this crucial chapter. Learn how to create a diet that not only nourishes but also protects your mind and body, ensuring a balanced and vibrant life. Embrace the wisdom within these pages and take the next step towards a healthier, happier you.

Refined Sugar

Why to Avoid:

Refined sugar, commonly found in sweets, sodas, and processed foods, can cause significant fluctuations in blood sugar levels, leading to mood swings and cognitive impairment.

Negative Effect on Mental Health and Overall Health:

Consuming high amounts of refined sugar leads to spikes and crashes in blood glucose levels. These rapid changes affect neurotransmitter function, crucial for mood regulation. When you consume sugar, it stimulates the release of dopamine, a neurotransmitter associated with pleasure. However, this rush is temporary and often followed by a sharp decline, which can contribute to feelings of anxiety and depression. Over time, the brain can become less responsive to dopamine, requiring more sugar to achieve the same pleasure, which creates a vicious cycle of addiction and mood disorders.

Beyond mental health, excessive sugar intake is a leading factor in the development of obesity, diabetes, and metabolic syndrome. These conditions not only deteriorate physical health but also have secondary effects on mental well-being. For instance, obesity and diabetes are associated with increased risks of depression and cognitive decline. Additionally, refined sugar promotes inflammation throughout the body, including the brain, which can exacerbate mental health issues.

Maximum Intake:

- No more than 25 grams (6 teaspoons) of added sugar per day for women and 36 grams (9 teaspoons) for men.

Potential Side Effects:

- Weight gain, insulin resistance, increased risk of cardiovascular disease, and dental cavities.

Trans Fats

Why to Avoid:

Trans fats are found in partially hydrogenated oils, often used in baked goods, fried foods, and margarine. They are detrimental to both mental and physical health.

Negative Effect on Mental Health and Overall Health:

Trans fats significantly increase inflammation and oxidative stress in the brain. This heightened inflammatory state can impair cognitive function and is associated with a higher risk of depression. Trans fats interfere with the proper functioning of cellular membranes and neurotransmitter activity, which are essential for maintaining optimal brain health. These disruptions can lead to a decline in mental sharpness and mood stability, making trans fats particularly harmful to mental health.

Beyond their effects on the brain, trans fats have severe implications for overall health. They raise levels of LDL (bad) cholesterol while simultaneously lowering levels of HDL (good) cholesterol. This imbalance increases the risk of developing heart disease, stroke, and type 2 diabetes. Furthermore, trans fats contribute to systemic inflammation, which can exacerbate a variety of chronic health conditions, further jeopardizing both physical and mental health.

Maximum Intake:

- Ideally, trans fat intake should be as low as possible, aiming for zero consumption.

Potential Side Effects:

- Increased risk of heart disease, systemic inflammation, and insulin resistance.

High-Fructose Corn Syrup (HFCS)

Why to Avoid:

HFCS is a sweetener found in many processed foods and beverages. It is associated with various negative health effects.

Negative Effect on Mental Health and Overall Health:

HFCS disrupts normal metabolism and can lead to insulin resistance. This metabolic disruption negatively affects brain function and mood regulation, contributing to mental health issues. High fructose intake is linked to impaired synaptic plasticity and memory function, which can hinder cognitive performance and learning capabilities. The detrimental impact of HFCS on brain health can exacerbate conditions such as anxiety and depression.

On a broader scale, HFCS consumption is associated with serious health problems like obesity and fatty liver disease. The high fructose content in HFCS promotes fat accumulation in the liver, leading to non-alcoholic fatty liver disease (NAFLD). Additionally, HFCS increases the risk of metabolic syndrome, a cluster of conditions that raise the risk of heart disease, stroke, and type 2 diabetes. The excessive intake of HFCS also contributes to systemic inflammation, further compounding its negative effects on overall health.

Maximum Intake:

- Similar to added sugars, limit HFCS intake to under 25-36 grams per day.

Potential Side Effects:

- Weight gain, liver damage, and increased risk of metabolic disorders.

Artificial Sweeteners

Why to Avoid:

Artificial sweeteners like aspartame, saccharin, and sucralose are often marketed as healthier alternatives to sugar due to their low-calorie content, but their impact on health is increasingly questioned.

Negative Effect on Mental Health and Overall Health:

Artificial sweeteners can have a detrimental effect on mental health. For instance, aspartame can cross the blood-brain barrier and affect neurotransmitter levels. This interference can potentially lead to headaches, mood changes, and cognitive dysfunction. Altered neurotransmitter levels can disrupt normal brain function, contributing to symptoms of anxiety and depression.

Furthermore, artificial sweeteners can negatively impact gut microbiota, the complex community of microorganisms in the digestive tract. A healthy gut microbiota is crucial for overall digestion and health, influencing everything from nutrient absorption to immune function. Disruption of this balance by artificial sweeteners can lead to digestive issues and broader health problems.

Chronic consumption of artificial sweeteners is also linked to metabolic derangements. Studies suggest that these sweeteners can lead to glucose intolerance, a precursor to metabolic syndrome and type 2 diabetes.

Maximum Intake:

- FDA-approved daily intake levels vary by sweetener but generally range from 50 mg/kg body weight for aspartame to 5 mg/kg for saccharin.

Potential Side Effects:

- Headaches, digestive issues, and possible long-term metabolic effects.

Processed Meats

Why to Avoid:

Processed meats such as sausages, hot dogs, and deli meats often contain high levels of nitrates, sodium, and preservatives.

Negative Effect on Mental Health and Overall Health:

Processed meats negatively affect mental health and overall health due to their content of harmful substances. Nitrates and nitrites, commonly used as preservatives in these meats, can convert into nitrosamines in the body. Nitrosamines are carcinogenic and may contribute to cognitive decline, potentially impacting brain health and increasing the risk of neurodegenerative diseases.

The high sodium content in processed meats is another major concern. Excessive sodium intake can lead to hypertension (high blood pressure), which adversely affects cardiovascular health. Hypertension is a risk factor for stroke and other cardiovascular diseases, which can have further implications for brain health and cognitive function.

Overall, regular consumption of processed meats is strongly linked to several chronic health conditions. These include an increased risk of colorectal cancer, heart disease, and type 2 diabetes. The carcinogenic potential of nitrosamines, combined with high sodium and saturated fat content, makes processed meats particularly detrimental to long-term health.

Maximum Intake:

- Limit processed meat consumption to less than one serving per week.

Potential Side Effects:

- Increased cancer risk, high blood pressure, and elevated risk of heart disease.

Alcohol

Why to Avoid:

While moderate alcohol consumption is sometimes touted for its potential health benefits, excessive drinking can have severe consequences for both mental and physical health. Understanding these risks is essential for making informed choices about alcohol consumption.

Negative Effect on Mental Health and Overall Health:

Alcohol acts as a central nervous system depressant, disrupting neurotransmitter balance and impairing brain function. This disruption can lead to mood disorders such as depression and anxiety, as well as cognitive impairments including memory loss and reduced executive function. Chronic alcohol use is particularly damaging, often resulting in brain shrinkage and damage to neuronal structures. This can exacerbate mental health issues and significantly impair cognitive abilities over time.

The physical health implications of excessive alcohol consumption are equally alarming. Alcohol abuse is a leading cause of liver disease, including fatty liver, hepatitis, and cirrhosis. These conditions can progress to liver failure, posing life-threatening risks. Additionally, heavy drinking increases the risk of cardiovascular problems such as hypertension, cardiomyopathy, and stroke. Alcohol is also a known risk factor for various cancers, including those of the mouth, throat, liver, breast, and colon.

Maximum Intake:

- Up to one drink per day for women and two drinks per day for men.

Potential Side Effects:

- Addiction, liver damage, and increased risk of mental health disorders.

Highly Caffeinated Drinks

Why to Avoid:

Energy drinks and excessive coffee consumption can lead to dangerously high caffeine intake, which can be harmful in large amounts. Understanding the potential risks associated with high caffeine consumption is crucial for maintaining both mental and physical health.

Negative Effect on Mental Health and Overall Health:

High caffeine intake can have several adverse effects on mental health. As a central nervous system stimulant, caffeine can lead to heightened anxiety, insomnia, and jitteriness. These effects are primarily due to caffeine's ability to increase cortisol levels, a stress hormone that can exacerbate feelings of stress and anxiety. Additionally, excessive caffeine consumption can interfere with sleep patterns, leading to chronic sleep deprivation, which further negatively impacts mental health by causing mood swings and cognitive impairment.

Physically, too much caffeine can lead to several health issues. It can cause heart palpitations and elevate blood pressure, increasing the risk of hypertension. Digestive issues such as acid reflux and stomach discomfort are also common side effects of high caffeine intake. Overconsumption of energy drinks, which often contain additional stimulants and high sugar levels, can compound these negative effects, posing even greater risks to overall health.

Maximum Intake:

- Up to 400 mg of caffeine per day (about four 8-ounce cups of coffee).

Potential Side Effects:

- Insomnia, increased heart rate, and digestive discomfort.

Foods High in Saturated Fats

Why to Avoid:

Foods such as fatty cuts of meat, butter, and full-fat dairy products are high in saturated fats, which can be detrimental to health.

Negative Effect on Mental Health and Overall Health:

Saturated fats have been shown to negatively impact brain health by increasing inflammation and oxidative stress. These fats can interfere with the structure and function of brain cells, potentially leading to cognitive decline and mood disorders. Diets high in saturated fats are linked to poorer memory and an increased risk of developing depression and anxiety. The inflammation caused by saturated fats can disrupt the balance of neurotransmitters, crucial for mood regulation and cognitive function.

Physically, saturated fats contribute to elevated levels of LDL (bad) cholesterol, which can lead to the buildup of plaque in arteries, increasing the risk of heart disease and stroke. High intake of saturated fats is also associated with obesity and metabolic syndrome, conditions that further exacerbate health problems. Excessive consumption of these fats can lead to increased blood pressure and insulin resistance, setting the stage for type 2 diabetes and cardiovascular issues.

Maximum Intake:

- Less than 10% of total daily calories should come from saturated fats.

Potential Side Effects:

- Heart disease, stroke, and elevated LDL cholesterol levels.

Excessive Sodium

Why to Avoid:

High sodium intake is common due to the prevalence of salt in processed and restaurant foods.

Negative Effect on Mental Health and Overall Health:

Excessive sodium can adversely affect mental health by contributing to high blood pressure, which reduces blood flow to the brain and increases the risk of stroke and cognitive decline. Elevated blood pressure can damage blood vessels, leading to decreased oxygen and nutrient delivery to brain cells, which impairs cognitive function and increases the risk of dementia. Furthermore, high sodium intake can cause fluid imbalance and dehydration, potentially impacting mood and cognitive abilities.

Overall, excessive sodium consumption is strongly linked to several severe health conditions. High sodium levels contribute to hypertension, which is a major risk factor for heart disease and stroke. The strain placed on the cardiovascular system by high blood pressure can lead to the development of heart disease and increase the risk of heart attacks. Additionally, excessive sodium intake can affect kidney function, leading to kidney damage and chronic kidney disease. The kidneys play a crucial role in regulating fluid balance and blood pressure, and excessive sodium can overwhelm their ability to function effectively.

Maximum Intake:

- Less than 2,300 mg per day, with an ideal limit of 1,500 mg for most adults.

Potential Side Effects:

- Hypertension, cardiovascular disease, and kidney damage.

Gluten (for Sensitive Individuals)

Why to Avoid:

For individuals with celiac disease or gluten sensitivity, gluten can cause severe health issues.

Negative Effect on Mental Health and Overall Health:

In gluten-sensitive individuals, the consumption of gluten can have a profound impact on mental health. Gluten can trigger inflammation and immune responses that negatively affect brain function, leading to symptoms such as brain fog, depression, and anxiety. These mental health issues arise because the immune response to gluten can cause inflammation in the brain and disrupt normal neurotransmitter activity.

Additionally, gluten can cause significant damage to the intestinal lining in individuals with celiac disease or gluten sensitivity. This damage impairs the absorption of essential nutrients, leading to various health problems, including nutrient deficiencies. Poor nutrient absorption can exacerbate mental health issues and contribute to overall physical health decline.

Overall, gluten sensitivity or celiac disease can lead to a range of digestive issues, such as abdominal pain, bloating, diarrhea, and constipation. Long-term gluten consumption in sensitive individuals increases the risk of developing autoimmune diseases, as the immune system continually reacts to the presence of gluten, leading to chronic inflammation and potential damage to other organs.

Maximum Intake:

- Gluten should be completely avoided by those with celiac disease or gluten sensitivity.

Potential Side Effects:

- Inflammatory responses, gastrointestinal distress, and nutrient malabsorption.

Understanding which nutrition to avoid is a critical step in optimizing your mental and physical health. By steering clear of refined sugar, trans fats, high-fructose corn syrup, artificial sweeteners, processed meats, alcohol, highly caffeinated drinks, foods high in saturated fats, excessive sodium and gluten, you can significantly reduce your risk of developing a myriad of health issues. These harmful substances can wreak havoc on your body, contributing to mood disorders, cognitive decline, and various chronic diseases. Making informed choices about what you eat empowers you to take control of your health, leading to a more balanced and vibrant life.

As you continue this journey toward better mental health, it's important to recognize that what you consume is only part of the equation. Equally vital is how well your body processes and utilizes the nutrients from the foods you eat. This brings us to the fascinating topic of gut health. In this next chapter, we will discover the intricate connection between your digestive system and your brain. You'll learn how a healthy gut can enhance your mood, boost cognitive function, and even alleviate symptoms of anxiety and depression. Stay tuned to discover practical tips and dietary strategies that will help you nurture your gut and, in turn, support a healthier, happier life.

Gut Health and Its Impact on Mental Well-Being

Why Gut Health Is Important

Gut health is a crucial aspect of overall well-being, significantly influencing both physical and mental health. The gut, often referred to as the "second brain," houses a complex community of trillions of microorganisms, collectively known as the gut microbiota. These microorganisms play a vital role in various bodily functions, including digestion, immune response, and the production of essential nutrients. However, one of the most fascinating aspects of gut health is its impact on mental well-being through the gut-brain axis.

The gut-brain axis is a bidirectional communication system linking the central nervous system (the brain and spinal cord) with the enteric nervous system (the network of neurons governing the gastrointestinal tract). This communication occurs via neural, hormonal, and immunological pathways, allowing the gut and brain to influence each other's functions.

Understanding this intricate relationship opens up exciting possibilities for enhancing mental health through better gut health. Did you know that the gut produces about 95% of the body's serotonin, a key neurotransmitter that regulates mood, sleep, and appetite? An imbalance in the gut microbiota can lead to a decrease in serotonin levels, potentially contributing to conditions like depression and anxiety. This is just one example of how closely linked our gut health is to our mental well-being.

Moreover, the gut microbiota helps modulate the body's immune response. Chronic inflammation, often a result of poor gut health, has been implicated in a variety of mental health disorders, including depression and schizophrenia. By maintaining a healthy gut, we can reduce inflammation and potentially improve our mental health.

Neurotransmitter Production

One of the most fascinating and impactful mechanisms of gut health on mental well-being is neurotransmitter production. The gut microbiota, a complex community of microorganisms residing in the digestive tract, plays a crucial role in the production of key neurotransmitters, including serotonin, dopamine, and gamma-aminobutyric acid (GABA). These neurotransmitters are essential for regulating mood, anxiety, and cognitive functions.

Serotonin, often referred to as the "feel-good" neurotransmitter, is a primary regulator of mood, emotion, and sleep. Remarkably, about 90% of the body's serotonin is produced in the gut, underscoring the importance of gut health in maintaining mental stability. When the gut microbiota is balanced and healthy, serotonin production is optimized, contributing to feelings of well-being and happiness. Conversely, an imbalanced gut can lead to decreased serotonin levels, potentially resulting in mood disorders such as depression and anxiety.

Dopamine, another vital neurotransmitter, is involved in reward, motivation, and pleasure. The gut microbiota influences dopamine production, which affects not only mood and motivation but also cognitive functions such as learning and memory. An unhealthy gut can disrupt dopamine synthesis, leading to cognitive impairments and reduced motivation.

GABA, a neurotransmitter that inhibits neural activity, helps to calm the nervous system and reduce anxiety. The gut microbiota's role in producing GABA highlights the gut-brain axis's importance in managing stress and anxiety levels. A balanced gut microbiome can enhance GABA production, promoting relaxation and reducing anxiety symptoms. Conversely, gut dysbiosis, an imbalance in the microbial community, can diminish GABA levels, contributing to heightened anxiety and stress.

Immune System Modulation

A significant portion of the immune system resides in the gut, making it a central player in maintaining overall health and particularly in modulating immune responses. The gut-associated lymphoid tissue (GALT) constitutes a large part of the body's immune system, housing around 70% of immune cells. These immune cells interact continuously with the gut microbiota, a diverse community of microorganisms that plays a crucial role in immune system regulation.

The gut microbiota helps maintain immune homeostasis by training the immune system to differentiate between harmful and harmless entities. This process is essential for preventing overreactions to non-threatening substances, which can lead to allergies and autoimmune disorders. The gut microbiota produces short-chain fatty acids (SCFAs) like butyrate, propionate, and acetate through the fermentation of dietary fibers. These SCFAs have anti-inflammatory properties and help modulate the activity of immune cells, reducing systemic inflammation.

Chronic inflammation, often a result of poor gut health, has been linked to various mental health disorders, including depression and anxiety. Inflammation can affect the brain by altering neurotransmitter systems, reducing neuroplasticity, and disrupting the blood-brain barrier. Pro-inflammatory cytokines, which are signaling molecules released by immune cells, can cross into the brain and influence mood regulation and cognitive functions.

The bidirectional communication between the gut and the brain, known as the gut-brain axis, highlights the importance of gut health in modulating the immune system and maintaining mental well-being. By nurturing a healthy gut microbiota through a balanced diet, probiotics, and lifestyle choices, it is possible to support immune homeostasis and reduce chronic inflammation, thus promoting better mental health.

Nutrient Synthesis

Gut bacteria play an essential role in synthesizing vital nutrients, making them indispensable for both brain function and overall health. These microorganisms contribute to the production of B vitamins and vitamin K, which are crucial for numerous bodily functions, including the maintenance of a healthy brain.

B vitamins, including B6, B12, and folate, are synthesized by gut bacteria and are critical for brain function. These vitamins are involved in the synthesis of neurotransmitters such as serotonin, dopamine, and gamma-aminobutyric acid (GABA), which regulate mood, sleep, and cognitive processes. B12 and folate are required for the methylation cycle, a biochemical process crucial for DNA repair and neurotransmitter production.

Vitamin K, another nutrient synthesized by gut bacteria, is essential for brain health. It plays a role in the synthesis of sphingolipids, a class of lipids found in high concentrations in brain cell membranes. Sphingolipids are involved in cell signaling and the protection of brain cells from oxidative stress. Therefore, vitamin K deficiency can impair cognitive function and increase the risk of neurodegenerative diseases.

In addition to synthesizing these essential vitamins, gut bacteria assist in the digestion and absorption of nutrients that support brain health. For example, the fermentation of dietary fibers by gut bacteria produces short-chain fatty acids (SCFAs) like butyrate, which have anti-inflammatory effects and promote a healthy gut lining.

The gut microbiota also aids in the absorption of minerals such as magnesium, zinc, and iron, which are vital for cognitive function and mood regulation. By maintaining a balanced gut microbiota through a diet rich in prebiotics, probiotics, and fiber, individuals can enhance nutrient synthesis and absorption, thereby supporting brain health and overall well-being.

Short-Chain Fatty Acids (SCFAs)

The fermentation of dietary fibers by gut bacteria produces short-chain fatty acids (SCFAs) such as butyrate, propionate, and acetate, which play a crucial role in maintaining both gut and brain health. These SCFAs not only serve as essential energy sources for colon cells but also possess anti-inflammatory properties that can protect the brain from inflammation-related damage.

Butyrate, one of the most studied SCFAs, is particularly beneficial for gut health. It serves as the primary energy source for colonocytes, the cells lining the colon, promoting their growth and repair. A healthy gut lining ensures effective nutrient absorption and prevents harmful pathogens from entering the bloodstream. Beyond the gut, butyrate exhibits neuroprotective effects. It can cross the blood-brain barrier and has been shown to enhance brain-derived neurotrophic factor (BDNF) levels, which support the survival and growth of neurons. Additionally, butyrate's anti-inflammatory properties help reduce neuroinflammation, a condition linked to various mental health disorders, including depression and Alzheimer's disease.

Propionate and acetate, the other significant SCFAs, also contribute to gut and brain health. Propionate has been shown to regulate glucose production and enhance insulin sensitivity, which is beneficial for overall metabolic health. This regulation can indirectly support brain health, as metabolic disorders like diabetes are associated with cognitive decline. Acetate, on the other hand, plays a role in appetite regulation and lipid metabolism, helping maintain a healthy weight and reducing the risk of obesity-related cognitive impairments.

The anti-inflammatory properties of SCFAs are critical in protecting the brain from inflammation-related damage. Chronic Inflammation is a known risk factor for neurodegenerative diseases and mental health disorders. SCFAs can modulate the immune system, reducing the production of pro-inflammatory cytokines and promoting the release of anti-inflammatory molecules. This modulation helps maintain a balanced immune response, protecting brain cells from chronic inflammatory damage.

By maintaining a diet rich in dietary fibers, individuals can support the production of SCFAs and promote overall gut and brain health. Foods such as fruits, vegetables, legumes, and whole grains are excellent sources of dietary fibers that foster a healthy gut microbiota, ultimately enhancing the production of beneficial SCFAs.

HPA Axis Regulation

The hypothalamic-pituitary-adrenal (HPA) axis is crucial for managing the body's stress response. The gut microbiota plays a significant role in regulating HPA axis activity, thereby influencing stress levels and anxiety. When the gut microbiota is balanced, it can help modulate the release of cortisol, the primary stress hormone, maintaining a stable response to stress. Conversely, an imbalanced gut microbiota can lead to dysregulation of the HPA axis, resulting in elevated cortisol levels and heightened stress and anxiety. This gut-brain interaction underscores the importance of a healthy microbiota for mental well-being. By maintaining a diet rich in prebiotics and probiotics, individuals can support a healthy gut microbiome, promoting optimal HPA axis function and reducing the impact of stress and anxiety on the body. Foods such as yogurt, kefir, and fiber-rich vegetables are beneficial in nurturing a healthy gut environment.

Given the intricate connection between gut health and mental well-being, maintaining a healthy gut microbiota is essential for promoting both physical and mental health. This can be achieved through a balanced diet rich in fiber, prebiotics, and probiotics, as well as lifestyle factors such as regular exercise and stress management.

Probiotic Supplements for Mental and Overall Health

The difference between pre and probiotics

Understanding the distinction between prebiotics and probiotics is essential for optimizing gut health and, consequently, mental well-being. Both play crucial roles in maintaining a healthy gut microbiome, but they function differently. Prebiotics provide the necessary nourishment to support the growth and activity of beneficial bacteria, while probiotics are the beneficial bacteria themselves. Together, they create a synergistic relationship that enhances gut health and promotes overall well-being.

Probiotics are live microorganisms that, when consumed in adequate amounts, confer health benefits on the host. These beneficial bacteria help maintain the balance of gut flora, aiding in digestion, boosting the immune system, and potentially enhancing mental health. Common sources of probiotics include fermented foods like yogurt, kefir, sauerkraut, kimchi, and certain types of cheese. Probiotic supplements are also available, often containing strains like Lactobacillus and Bifidobacterium.

Prebiotics, on the other hand, are non-digestible food components that promote the growth and activity of beneficial bacteria in the gut. Essentially, prebiotics serve as food for probiotics, helping them to thrive and maintain a balanced gut environment. Prebiotics include specific types of fiber such as inulin, fructooligosaccharides (FOS), and galactooligosaccharides (GOS).

Inulin is a type of soluble fiber found in a variety of plants. It can be found in foods such as chicory root, garlic, onions, leeks, asparagus, and bananas. Inulin is beneficial for the gut microbiome as it ferments in the colon, producing short-chain fatty acids that nourish colon cells and support gut health.

Fructooligosaccharides (FOS) are another form of prebiotic fiber that can be found in foods like garlic, onions, leeks, asparagus, bananas, and Jerusalem artichokes. FOS helps promote the growth of beneficial bacteria, improving digestive health and enhancing nutrient absorption.

Galactooligosaccharides (GOS) are prebiotic fibers found in foods like legumes, beans, and certain root vegetables. GOS promotes the growth of beneficial bacteria, particularly Bifidobacteria, in the gut, supporting overall gut health and improving immune function.

While probiotics introduce beneficial bacteria into the gut, prebiotics nourish and support these microorganisms, ensuring their survival and effectiveness. Together, they create a synergistic effect, enhancing gut health more effectively than either could alone. Incorporating both into your diet can lead to improved digestion, a stronger immune system, and better mental health through the gut-brain axis.

Next, we will discover the top 10 probiotics, exploring their specific benefits, sources, and how they can contribute to a healthier gut and improved mental well-being. Stay tuned to discover how these powerful microorganisms can transform your health.

Incorporating these probiotics into your daily routine can help maintain a healthy gut microbiota, which in turn supports mental well-being and overall health. However, it is important to consult with a healthcare professional before starting any new supplement regimen to ensure it is appropriate for your individual health needs.

Lactobacillus rhamnosus GG

Effect on Health: *Lactobacillus rhamnosus* GG is known for its ability to survive stomach acid and colonize the gut. It enhances the gut barrier function, modulates the immune system, and has been shown to reduce anxiety and depression symptoms by influencing GABA receptor expression in the brain.

Daily Intake: 10-20 billion CFUs (colony-forming units).

Potential Side Effects: Mild digestive discomfort, such as gas or bloating, which usually subsides with continued use.

Bifidobacterium longum

Effect on Health: Bifidobacterium longum helps reduce inflammation and supports the gut barrier. It has been associated with reduced symptoms of anxiety and improved cognitive function, potentially through its anti-inflammatory effects and influence on tryptophan metabolism, which is crucial for serotonin production.

Daily Intake: 1-10 billion CFUs.

Potential Side Effects: Generally well-tolerated, but some may experience mild bloating or gas.

Lactobacillus helveticus R0052

Effect on Health: This strain is effective in reducing stress and anxiety by modulating the gut-brain axis. It can lower cortisol levels, a hormone associated with stress, and improve overall gut health by enhancing gut barrier integrity and reducing inflammation.

Daily Intake: 1-10 billion CFUs.

Potential Side Effects: Minimal, with occasional mild digestive discomfort.

Bifidobacterium bifidum

Effect on Health: *Bifidobacterium bifidum* supports the immune system, reduces gut inflammation, and enhances nutrient absorption. It has been linked to improved mood and cognitive function by maintaining a balanced gut microbiota and supporting neurotransmitter production.

Daily Intake: 1-10 billion CFUs.

Potential Side Effects: Mild gas or bloating in some individuals.

Lactobacillus plantarum

Effect on Health: *Lactobacillus plantarum* is known for its robust anti-inflammatory properties and ability to enhance gut barrier function. It has been shown to reduce symptoms of depression and anxiety by promoting the production of serotonin and other mood-regulating neurotransmitters.

Daily Intake: 10-20 billion CFUs.

Potential Side Effects: Generally well-tolerated, but some may experience minor digestive issues initially.

Bifidobacterium lactis

Effect on Health: *Bifidobacterium lactis* supports digestion, enhances the immune response, and helps reduce gastrointestinal discomfort. It has been associated with improved mood and mental clarity by supporting a healthy gut microbiome and reducing systemic inflammation.

Daily Intake: 1-10 billion CFUs.

Potential Side Effects: Rare, with possible mild digestive discomfort.

Saccharomyces boulardii

Effect on Health: This probiotic yeast helps restore gut flora balance, particularly during and after antibiotic use. It can reduce gut inflammation and support the production of short-chain fatty acids, which benefit brain health and cognitive function.

Daily Intake: 5-10 billion CFUs.

Potential Side Effects: Mild constipation or thirst in some individuals.

Lactobacillus casei

Effect on Health: *Lactobacillus casei* aids in digestion and reduces gut inflammation. It has been shown to improve mood and reduce anxiety by enhancing the production of serotonin and modulating the immune response.

Daily Intake: 10-20 billion CFUs.

Potential Side Effects: Mild digestive discomfort, such as gas or bloating.

Bifidobacterium breve

Effect on Health: *Bifidobacterium breve* helps maintain a healthy gut microbiota, reduces inflammation, and supports digestion. It has been linked to improved mental health by enhancing the gut-brain axis communication and supporting neurotransmitter balance.

Daily Intake: 1-10 billion CFUs.

Potential Side Effects: Generally well-tolerated, with occasional mild digestive issues.

Lactobacillus acidophilus

Effect on Health: *Lactobacillus acidophilus* supports digestion, boosts the immune system, and enhances nutrient absorption. It has been associated with improved mood and reduced anxiety by promoting a balanced gut microbiota and supporting serotonin production.

Daily Intake: 10-20 billion CFUs.

Potential Side Effects: Mild digestive discomfort, such as gas or bloating, may occur initially.

Supplement Plan to Conquer Anxiety

Anxiety is a complex condition influenced by various factors, including nutritional imbalances and deficiencies. To address anxiety effectively, a comprehensive supplement plan incorporating herbal supplements, nootropics, and probiotics can be beneficial. Here, we provide a detailed advisory with daily intakes and recommendations on when to take each supplement.

Herbal Supplements

Ashwagandha

- **Daily Intake:** 300 mg twice daily

- **When to Take:** Morning and evening

Rhodiola Rosea

- **Daily Intake:** 200 mg once daily

- **When to Take:** Morning

Chamomile

- **Daily Intake:** 300-400 mg three times daily

- **When to Take:** Morning, afternoon, and evening

Nootropics

L-Theanine

- **Daily Intake:** 200 mg daily

- **When to Take:** Morning

Phosphatidylserine

- **Daily Intake:** 300 mg daily

- **When to Take:** Evening

Magnesium L-Threonate

- **Daily Intake:** 1,000 mg daily

- **When to Take:** Evening

Probiotics

Lactobacillus rhamnosus

- **Daily Intake:** 10 billion CFU daily

- **When to Take:** Morning

Bifidobacterium longum

- **Daily Intake:** 10 billion CFU daily

- **When to Take:** Morning

Daily Intake Plan Reducing Anxiety

Time of Day	Supplements
Morning	Ashwagandha, Rhodiola Rosea, L-Theanine, Lactobacillus rhamnosus, Bifidobacterium longum, Chamomile
Afternoon	Chamomile
Evening	Ashwagandha, Phosphatidylserine, Magnesium L-Threonate, Chamomile

Supplement Plan to Conquer Depression

Depression is a multifaceted condition that can be influenced by various factors, including nutritional imbalances and deficiencies. A comprehensive supplement plan incorporating herbal supplements, nootropics, and probiotics can be beneficial in addressing depression. Below is a detailed advisory with daily intakes and recommendations on when to take each supplement.

Herbal Supplements

St. John's Wort

- **Daily Intake:** 300 mg three times daily

- **When to Take:** Morning, afternoon, and evening

Saffron

- **Daily Intake:** 30 mg daily

- **When to Take:** Morning

Lavender

- **Daily Intake:** 80 mg twice daily

- **When to Take:** Morning and evening

Nootropics

SAM-e

- **Daily Intake:** 400 mg twice daily

- **When to Take:** Morning and afternoon

Acetyl-L-Carnitine (ALCAR)

- **Daily Intake:** 1,000 mg daily

- **When to Take:** Morning

Omega-3 Fatty Acids (EPA/DHA)

- **Daily Intake:** 1,000 mg daily

- **When to Take:** Morning

Probiotics

Lactobacillus helveticus R0052

- **Daily Intake:** 10 billion CFU daily

- **When to Take:** Morning

Bifidobacterium bifidum

- **Daily Intake:** 10 billion CFU daily

- **When to Take:** Morning

Daily Intake Plan Conquering Depression

Time of Day	Supplements
Morning	St. John's Wort, Saffron, Lavender, SAM-e, Acetyl-L-Carnitine, Omega-3 Fatty Acids, Lactobacillus helveticus R0052, Bifidobacterium bifidum
Afternoon	St. John's Wort, SAM-e
Evening	St. John's Wort, Lavender

Supplement Plan to Relieve Stress

Stress is a pervasive condition that affects mental and physical well-being. Addressing stress effectively requires a comprehensive approach, including the use of herbal supplements, nootropics, and probiotics. Here is a detailed advisory with daily intakes and recommendations on when to take each supplement.

Herbal Supplements

Holy Basil (Tulsi)

- **Daily Intake:** 500 mg twice daily

- **When to Take:** Morning and evening

Ashwagandha

- **Daily Intake:** 300 mg twice daily

- **When to Take:** Morning and evening

Passionflower

- **Daily Intake:** 400 mg three times daily

- **When to Take:** Morning, afternoon, and evening

Nootropics

L-Theanine

- **Daily Intake:** 200 mg daily

- **When to Take:** Morning

Rhodiola Rosea

- **Daily Intake:** 200 mg once daily

- **When to Take:** Morning

Phosphatidylserine

- **Daily Intake:** 300 mg daily

- **When to Take:** Evening

Probiotics

Lactobacillus rhamnosus GG

- **Daily Intake:** 10 billion CFU daily

- **When to Take:** Morning

Bifidobacterium longum

- **Daily Intake:** 10 billion CFU daily

- **When to Take:** Morning

Daily Intake Plan to Relieve Stress

Time of Day	Supplements
Morning	Holy Basil, Ashwagandha, Passionflower, L-Theanine, Rhodiola Rosea, Lactobacillus rhamnosus GG, Bifidobacterium longum
Afternoon	Passionflower
Evening	Holy Basil, Ashwagandha, Passionflower, Phosphatidylserine

Supplement Plan to Relieve Cognitive Dysfunction

Cognitive dysfunction, which encompasses issues with memory, focus, and mental clarity, can be alleviated through a strategic supplement plan. Incorporating herbal supplements, nootropics, and probiotics can significantly enhance cognitive function. Here is a detailed advisory with daily intakes and recommendations on when to take each supplement.

Herbal Supplements

Ginkgo Biloba

- **Daily Intake:** 120-240 mg daily

- **When to Take:** Morning

Bacopa Monnieri

- **Daily Intake:** 300 mg twice daily

- **When to Take:** Morning and evening

Rhodiola Rosea

- **Daily Intake:** 200 mg once daily

- **When to Take:** Morning

Nootropics

Alpha-GPC (L-Alpha glycerylphosphorylcholine)

- **Daily Intake:** 300 mg twice daily

- **When to Take:** Morning and afternoon

Lion's Mane Mushroom

- **Daily Intake:** 500 mg twice daily

- **When to Take:** Morning and evening

Acetyl-L-Carnitine (ALCAR)

- **Daily Intake:** 500 mg twice daily

- **When to Take:** Morning and afternoon

Probiotics

Lactobacillus plantarum

- **Daily Intake:** 10 billion CFU daily

- **When to Take:** Morning

Bifidobacterium bifidum

- **Daily Intake:** 10 billion CFU daily

- **When to Take:** Morning

Daily intake plan to Relieve Cognitive Dysfunction

Time of Day	Supplements
Morning	Ginkgo Biloba, Bacopa Monnieri, Rhodiola Rosea, Alpha-GPC, Lion's Mane Mushroom, Acetyl-L-Carnitine, Lactobacillus plantarum, Bifidobacterium bifidum
Afternoon	Alpha-GPC, Acetyl-L-Carnitine
Evening	Bacopa Monnieri, Lion's Mane Mushroom

Guidelines for supplement plans

Start with the recommended daily intakes and monitor your body's response over the first few weeks. Adjust dosages as necessary under the guidance of a healthcare professional. For optimal results, this plan should be followed consistently for at least 3-6 months.

Taking supplements for an extended period, such as three months or more, is crucial for several reasons. First, many supplements, especially herbal and nootropic ones, require time to build up in your system and exert their full effects. Initial improvements may be subtle, with more significant changes becoming evident over time. Consistent use allows the body to adapt and respond to the beneficial compounds, gradually improving mental health and cognitive function.

Secondly, chronic conditions like anxiety, depression, stress, and cognitive dysfunction often develop over extended periods and, likewise, require sustained intervention to address the underlying imbalances effectively. A few weeks of supplementation may not be sufficient to bring about lasting change, whereas a longer duration helps ensure that the body has adequate time to heal and rebalance.

Periodic evaluations with a healthcare provider can help determine if continued supplementation is needed based on improvements and overall well-being. This ongoing assessment ensures that the supplement plan remains tailored to your individual needs and that any necessary adjustments are made to optimize benefits.

Combining these herbal supplements, nootropics, and probiotics with a balanced diet can create a synergistic effect, promoting mental health and reducing anxiety, depression, stress, or cognitive dysfunction. This holistic approach leverages the benefits of each supplement to support your journey towards a calmer, more balanced state of mind. Maintaining this regimen over several months ensures a more profound and lasting impact on your overall mental well-being.

Dear Reader,

As you reach the end of this book, I hope you feel empowered with knowledge and ready to take proactive steps toward better mental health. I've shared insights on how nutritional supplements can play a significant role in supporting your journey. However, it's crucial to remember that supplements are not a cure-all.

Mental health is deeply personal and complex, often requiring the expertise of professionals. If you are struggling with anxiety, depression, stress, or cognitive dysfunction, I urge you to seek help from a qualified mental health professional like a psychotherapist or psychiatrist. They can provide tailored strategies and treatments that address your unique needs.

Think of supplements as companions on your mental health journey. They can enhance and complement the professional care you receive, adding a layer of support that works in harmony with therapy or medication. By combining professional guidance with the right nutritional support, you can create a robust, holistic approach to mental well-being.

The beauty of this approach lies in its comprehensiveness. While a therapist helps you navigate your thoughts and emotions, supplements can provide the physical foundation your brain needs to function optimally. Together, they create a balanced path toward a healthier, happier you.

Thank you for allowing me to share this journey with you. Take care of yourself, reach out for the support you need, and embrace the small, daily steps that lead to lasting well-being.

Warm regards,

Samuel Hayes